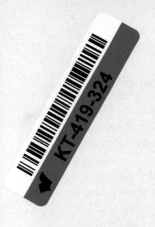
KT-419-324

CDU

OXFORD MEDICAL PUBLICATIONS

Stroke:

past, present, and future

Oxford University Press makes no representation, express or implied, that the drug dosages in this book are correct. Readers must therefore always check the product information and clinical procedures with the most up-to-date published product information and data sheets provided by the manufacturers and the most recent codes of conduct and safety regulations. The authors and the publishers do not accept responsibility or legal liability for any errors in the text or for the misuse or misapplication of material in this work.

Stroke:

past, present, and future

EDITED BY

W.W. HOLLAND

Chairman of Research and Development Committee
The Stroke Association

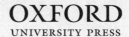

OXFORD
UNIVERSITY PRESS

Great Clarendon Street, Oxford OX2 6DP

Oxford University Press is a department of the University of Oxford.
It furthers the University's objective of excellence in research, scholarship,
and education by publishing worldwide in

Oxford New York

Athens Auckland Bangkok Bogotá Buenos Aires Calcutta
Cape Town Chennai Dar es Salaam Delhi Florence Hong Kong Istanbul
Karachi Kuala Lumpur Madrid Melbourne Mexico City Mumbai
Nairobi Paris São Paulo Singapore Taipei Tokyo Toronto Warsaw

with associated companies in
Berlin Ibadan

Oxford is a registered trade mark of Oxford University Press
in the UK and in certain other countries

Published in the United States
by Oxford University Press Inc., New York

© Oxford University Press, 2000

The moral rights of the author have been asserted
Database right Oxford University Press (maker)

First published 2000

All rights reserved. No part of this publication may be reproduced,
stored in a retrieval system, or transmitted, in any form or by any means,
without the prior permission in writing of Oxford University Press,
or as expressly permitted by law, or under terms agreed with the appropriate
reprographics rights organization. Enquiries concerning reproduction
outside the scope of the above should be sent to the Rights Department,
Oxford University Press, at the address above

You must not circulate this book in any other binding or cover
and you must impose this same condition on any acquirer

A catalogue record for this title is available
from the British library

Library of Congress Cataloging in Publication Data
(Data available)

1 3 5 7 9 10 8 6 4 2

ISBN 0 19 263152 7

Typeset by Newgen Imaging Systems (P) Ltd., Chennai, India
Printed in Great Britain on acid-free paper by
Biddles Ltd, Guildford & King's Lynn

Preface

This scientific conference inaugurates our centenary year. The Stroke Association is very proud of the research it has supported over the years. Many of the advances in prevention, acute care, and rehabilitation in the management of stroke can be linked to the research sponsored by our Association. Stroke is a terrible affliction but its incidence has diminished in the past 10 years, survival has improved, but most dramatically there has been significant improvement in the quality of life and levels of disability of those who survive the initial period due to improvements in treatment and care.

We must, however, not rest on our laurels. The quality, scope, and amount of research on stroke have increased tremendously in recent years. But there are innumerable gaps in our knowledge which, if filled, could be of immeasurable help both in the prevention and treatment of stroke.

We hope that this meeting, while celebrating our success, will also give encouragement for future efforts and increased resources to fulfil our aims.

Professor Walter Holland
Chairman of Research and Development Committee
The Stroke Association

Contents

Section 5: Imaging

Section 6: Therapy and rehabilitation

Section 7: Stroke and stroke care

List of contributors

Dr Ann Ashburn
MSc Course Coordinator/Senior Lecturer in Rehabilitation, Southampton General Hospital

Dr John Bamford
Consultant Neurologist and Cerebrovascular Physician, St James' University Hospital, Leeds

Professor Philip Bath
Professor of Stroke Medicine, Nottingham City Hospital

Professor John C. Brocklehurst
Emeritus Professor of Geriatric Medicine, University of Manchester

Professor Martin M. Brown
Professor of Stroke Medicine, Institute of Neurology, London

Dr Avril Drummond
Senior Occupational Therapist/Research Officer, University of Nottingham

Professor Shah Ebrahim
Professor of Epidemiology of Ageing, MRC Health Services Research Collaboration, University of Bristol

Professor Pam Enderby
Chair of Community Rehabilitation, Centre for Ageing and Rehabilitation Studies, University of Sheffield

Alison Halliday
Consultant in Vascular Surgery, Epsom General Hospital and St George's Hospital, London

Professor Walter W. Holland
Emeritus Professor of Public Health Medicine, University of London; Chairman of Research and Development Committee, The Stroke Association

Dr Allan House
Consultant and Senior Lecturer in Liaison Psychiatry, Department of Psychiatry, University of Leeds

Professor Kay-Tee Khaw
Professor of Clinical Gerontology, Addenbrooke's Hospital, Cambridge

Dr Peter Langhorne
Senior Lecturer in Geriatric Medicine, Academic Section of Geriatric Medicine, University of Glasgow

Dr Hugh S. Markus
Reader in Neurology, Guy's, King's, and St Thomas' School of Medicine and Institute of Psychiatry, London

Professor John Marshall
Chairman of Executive Committee, The Stroke Association

Professor Paul M. Matthews
Consultant in Neurology, Centre for Functional Magnetic Resonance Imaging of the Brain, Department of Clinical Neurology, University of Oxford, Oxford

Professor A. David Mendelow
Consultant in Neurosurgery, Newcastle General Hospital, University of Newcastle

Dr Hirofumi Nakayama
Secretary General of the Japan Stroke Association, Department of Internal Medicine, Osaka National Hospital, Japan

Professor John F. Potter
Division of Medicine for the Elderly, The Glenfield Hospital, Leicester

Judith Redfern
Research Fellow, MRC Health Services Research Collaboration, Royal Free and University College Medical School

Dr Helen Rodgers
Senior Lecturer in Stroke Medicine, University of Newcastle upon Tyne

Professor Martin Severs
Professor in Elderly Health Care, Queen Alexandra Hospital, Portsmouth

Professor Ray Tallis
Professor of Geriatric Medicine, Hope Hospital, Salford

Dr Dafydd J. Thomas
Consultant in Neurology, St Mary's Hospital, London

Professor Jan van Gijn
Professor of Neurology, University Department of Neurology, Utrecht, The Netherlands

Dr Graham S. Venables
Consultant in Neurology, Royal Hallamshire Hospital, Sheffield

Professor Charles P. Warlow
Professor of Medical Neurology, Department of Clinical Neurosciences, University of Edinburgh

Dr Charles Wolfe
Reader in Public Health Medicine, Guy's, King's, and St Thomas' Hospitals School of Medicine, London

1

How it was

PROFESSOR JOHN MARSHALL

Chairman of Executive Committee
The Stroke Association

Before the establishment of the National Health Service in 1948, hospitals in the UK were either supported by voluntary contributions – the voluntary hospitals – or run by the local authority – the municipal hospitals. A resident medical officer in a voluntary hospital, with an eye to his future, would do everything in his power to avoid admitting a stroke patient to one of the consultants' beds. Patients with strokes were to go to the municipal hospital. Why? Because 'there was nothing to be done'. Such was the attitude towards people with stroke. It is true that there was at that time no specific treatment for acute stroke, but because of this general measures were neglected; aspiration, chest infection, dehydration, urinary infection, and bed sores took their toll.

What brought about the change? It might be thought that the introduction of cerebral angiography by Moniz in 1927[1] with his description of occlusion of the cervical segment of the carotid artery was the stimulus, but this was not the case. Angiography was used in the diagnosis of aneurysms and to detect the 'blush' produced by a meningioma or the 'malignant circulation' of a glioma, but it was not applied to atherosclerotic vascular disease. Indeed, its use in vascular disease was strongly discouraged because it was said to carry significant risk of causing a stroke.

The change in attitude to stroke came about following the introduction of anticoagulants in the treatment of acute coronary artery occlusion with the demonstration of their value by controlled trials. It was argued that what was beneficial for coronary artery occlusion should also be of benefit for occlusion of a cerebral artery. Towards the end of the 1950s a number of single case reports and reports of uncontrolled series were published, conveying uncritical approval. The first randomized controlled trials of anticoagulants in acute stroke and in long-term secondary prevention published in 1960[2,3] were not so encouraging. They brought to light a problem not encountered with coronary occlusion, namely, the risk of cerebral haemorrhage. One must remember that these trials were carried out before the introduction of the CT scan; exclusion of cerebral haemorrhage as the cause of a stroke had to be by clinical criteria alone, which proved to be less than reliable.

Today's stroke physician would not countenance giving anticoagulants or, indeed, any other therapy to a patient with a stroke without first securing a CT scan, and rightly so. But the situation in the late 1950s was not as nerve wracking as it must appear to modern eyes. The CT scan had not been invented and so there was no feeling of managing patients under less than ideal conditions. Careful clinical assessment was the best tool available and was applied carefully and conscientiously.

Although anticoagulants proved to be a disappointment, they served a valuable purpose by arousing interest in stroke and making it a 'respectable' subject for those wishing to do research. This change in attitude was greatly encouraged by the introduction by Niels Lassen in 1955[4] of methods of measuring cerebral blood flow, first by krypton and then by xenon, which could be used in a clinical setting. The identification of cerebral blood flow phenomena such as luxury-perfusion, steal, and reverse steal (the Robin Hood phenomenon) greatly advanced our understanding of what happens to the cerebral circulation in stroke. It also called attention to the danger of lowering blood pressure in situations in which vascular reactivity has been damaged. An interesting feature of this surge of interest is that, although neurologists only dealt with one or two per cent of acute strokes, they led the research activity in the field. Activity in the field of rehabilitation, which is outside the scope of this chapter, was led by geriatricians.

Another important development was recognition of the importance of transient ischaemic attacks (TIAs). The clinical features were described in the 19th century but their significance as a harbinger of stroke was largely the result of the work, in the 1950s, of Miller Fisher, in particular his observation of transient occlusion of a retinal artery during an attack of amaurosis fugax.[5] These observations laid to rest the widely held view that TIAs were caused by vasospasm; the embolic origin of the great majority was firmly established. This in turn led to the recognition of internal carotid stenosis as a source of the emboli and, as its removal by the newly developed technique of endarterectomy was now possible, the use of surgery in this situation.

Thus in a very short period spanning not much more than a decade, stroke had changed from a completely neglected subject 'because there was nothing to be done', to one of active clinical management and intense research. Although none of the initial therapies was dramatically effective, the mortality of acute stroke began to fall. This was because interest in the patient and the condition led to better management of the long list of complications from which stroke patients previously died.

Parallel to the activity in the management of acute stroke, significant progress was being made in the identification of risk factors for stroke and in their prevention. This again was a spin-off from research in the field of coronary heart disease. The first prospective study of a community was started in Framingham, Massachusetts in 1954.[6] Its primary focus was heart disease but the importance of risk factors for stroke soon became available from its data. Hypertension was recognized as the most important risk factor for stroke followed by diabetes mellitus, hyperlipidaemia, cardiac abnormalities, cigarette smoking, and the oral contraceptive. The encouraging feature was that these factors were amenable to management. This led to campaigns to 'know your blood pressure', to stop smoking, etc., which have in turn led to a decline in the incidence of stroke.

The second half of the 20th century has been an exciting time for those working in the field of stroke. Those who embarked on it in the 1950s were entering a completely neglected and uncharted field. A conference such as this one would have been unthinkable at that time. It is interesting that it was the prospect of therapy rather than scientific or technological advances – valuable though these were – that spurred them on. That initial therapies were disappointing did not prove a deterrent. Appetites had been whetted, the bandwagon had started to roll, so that we can approach the end of the century and of the millennium with a feeling of satisfaction about what has been achieved and keen anticipation as to what the next millennium will bring.

References

1. Moniz, E., Lima, A., De Lacerda, R. (1927). Hemiplegics par thrombose de la carotide inteme. *Presse Med.*, **45**, 977–80.
2. Marshall, J., Shaw, D. A. (1960). Anticoagulant therapy in acute cerebrovascular accidents. A controlled trial. *Lancet*, **1**, 995–8.
3. Hill, A. B., Marshall, J., Shaw, D. A. (1960). A controlled clinical trial of long-term anticoagulant therapy in cerebrovascular disease. *Quart. J. Med.*, **29**, 597–609.

4. Lassen, N. A., Munck, O. (1955). The cerebral blood flow in man determined by the use of radioactive krypton. *Acta Physiol. Scand.*, **33**, 30–49.
5. Fisher, C. M. (1959). Observations of the fundus oculi in transient monocular blindness. *Neurology* (Minneap.), **9**, 333–47.
6. Kannel, W. B., Dawber, T. R., Cohen, M. E., McNamara, P. M. (1965). Vascular disease of the brain – epidemiological aspects: The Framingham study. *Am. J. Pub. Health*, **55**, 1355–66.

2   Stroke as it was

PROFESSOR J. C. BROCKLEHURST

Emeritus Professor of Geriatric Medicine
University of Manchester

This contribution discusses rehabilitation and the social aspects of stroke up to 1975. Early rehabilitation methods described in the 15th century by Coelius Auralianus included heat, hydrotherapy, weights, pulleys, and walking machines. By the early 19th century management had regressed to bleeding, blisters to the head, mustard cataplasms to the feet, stinging nettles, and sea bathing (Clarke, 1805). Electricity followed the development of Volta's battery in 1800 and had a varied career through the next 150 years. It was recommended by Clarke in 1805 (both sparks and shock), and was followed by 'galvanism to the head' (Pultiney Allison, 1864), 'faradism but never galvanism' (Charlton Bastion, 1875), 'absolutely no electricity' (Conybeare, 1929), and 'mild faradism' (Cecil and Foster Kennedy, 1943). Croton oil (1–2 drops) was popular for the bowels. Swallowing problems were addressed by Hilton Fagge and Pye Smith (1891) recommending the rectal administration of beef tea and milk. Massage and flannel next to the skin also had their advocates. Drugs included strychnine, quinine, iron, and potassium iodide. Cowslips (Gerard, 1597) sound safer!

Generally, however, after a few weeks in bed patients with relatives and carers were left to provide their own common-sense approach to recovery. Other stroke patients, however, were admitted to workhouse infirmaries and chronic sick wards where they remained in bed for the rest of their lives, developing horrific contractures.

It was in this setting that a systematic approach to rehabilitation began. In 1935, Dr Marjorie Warren (the 'mother' of geriatrics) took responsibility for the workhouse infirmary associated with the West Middlesex Hospital and developed a vigorous rehabilitation campaign for the 714 patients 'warehoused' there. This first involved obtaining chairs, clothes, and shoes. The simplest equipment she could devise was a board, 3" × 4" × 40", laid across the floor against the bottom legs of the iron bedstead. Seated facing the bottom of the bed and holding the bed-frame, the patients performed 'bed-end exercise' – a technique which continued until the introduction of King's Fund adjustable beds in the 1970s.

Several surveys in the 1940s indicated the massive problems of the chronic sick that had to be solved. Professor (later Sir) Arthur Thomson in his Goulstonian lectures to the Royal College of Physicians in 1949 described 50 institutions in the Birmingham region concerned with the reception of the elderly and chronic sick – a total of 5780 patients, 45% of whom were chronically ill – 23% of the males and 16% of the females with hemiplegia – two-thirds of them aged 70 and over. In the Western Road Infirmary there were 100 bedridden patients, plus 150 who were ambulant. He wrote:

In Western Road no masseuse (physiotherapist [PT]) had worked for years. There was a room reserved for physiotherapy but on the door was the notice 'Do not enter' and within, a heap of electrical apparatus, apparently in good order. Rehabilitation could not be attempted because there was no staff and all the day rooms were full of beds. There was no occupational or recreational therapy, but a few women patients knitted or did needlework. I never saw a man engage in any spontaneous activity in all the wards.[1]

It was in settings such as these that geriatric medicine began, evolving a system of progressive patient care – acute assessment, rehabilitation, and long-term care. Rehabilitation was centered on multidisciplinary teams of doctor, nurse, therapist, and social worker. Nurses were generally in short supply (Thomson had noted two nurses on duty in wards containing 70 patients), therapists had to be 'fought' for, and occupational therapists (OTs) were a gift from above. OTs were easier to get than PTs, the latter 'belonged to the surgeons, the former was nobody's baby'.[2] Almoners – later to become medical social workers – also became vital team members. The multidisciplinary team drew up and supervised individual and group therapy programmes for hemiplegic and other patients, supervised their progress, and prepared them for discharge.

Day hospitals were developed for post-discharge rehabilitation and treatment and for those never admitted (one-third of stroke survivors at two weeks according to one survey).[3] There was early emphasis on developing the non-affected limbs (the good carrying the bad, as in pulley exercises); posture that sagged to the sound side was often supported with a tripod walking stick and with a heavy caliper overcoming foot drop on the affected side and pain and contracture developing in the shoulder and arm. Awareness of the inherent dangers of this approach was expressed by Adams.[4]

The essentials of stroke rehabilitation were to prevent contracture, to concentrate in the early stages on the proximal muscle groups, to restore balance and confidence when moving, to avoid overuse of the good side at the expense of the hemiplegic limbs, and to strive, if necessary for months, to obtain a polished rhythmical gait and not accept too easily, or too readily, the stilted awkwardness of the 'traditional hobble'. As knowledge progressed about balance, body image, and neglect, so therapy became more specific and was finally revolutionized by the work, among others, of Bobath, Brunstrome, and Twitchell.[5] Speech therapists entered the rehabilitation team, their role extending beyond accelerating spontaneous return of language to giving hope, contact, someone to relate to, and guidance for relatives and carers as well as dysphasic patients themselves. Their role in assessment of swallowing was to come later. Valerie Eaton Griffiths in 1970 developed a system of using shifts of volunteers to provide hours of stimulation and participation every day for dysphasic patients at home, supplementing the speech therapist's twice or thrice weekly sessions.

Community interest was stimulated by relatives' conferences set up for in-patients (e.g. by formation of stroke clubs). Recreational and creative activities for those patients requiring long-term hospital stay were developed, and young disabled units on the lines of Cheshire Homes were mandated in the Chronically Sick and Disabled Person's Act of 1970.

References

1. Thomson, A. P. (1949). Problems of ageing and chronic sickness. *Br. Med. J.*, **ii**, 244–50, 300–5.
2. Matthews, D. A. (1984). Dr Marjorie Warren and the origin of British geriatrics. *J. Am. Geriat. Soc.*, **32**, 253–8.
3. Brocklehurst, J. C., Andrews, K., Morris, P., Richards, B. R., Laycock, P. L. (1978). Why admit stroke patients to hospital? *Age Aging*, **7**, 100–8.
4. Adams, G. F. (1971). Capacity after stroke. *Br. Med. J.*, **i**, 91–3.
5. Bobath, B. (1970). *Adult hemiplegia*. Heinemann, London.

Section 1

Epidemiology and primary prevention

3   Risk factors, causes, and distribution of stroke

PROFESSOR KAY-TEE KHAW

Professor of Clinical Gerontology
Addenbrooke's Hospital, Cambridge

Introduction

Stroke accounts for about 10% of all deaths in industrialized countries and is a leading cause of disability in the community. Since
stroke rates rise sharply with age, the increasing number of older
people in the population is of concern in terms of projected impact
of stroke. However, profound geographic and socio-economic variations and time trends in stroke rates suggest that stroke is a highly
preventable condition. There are substantial international variations
with men and women in the highest rate countries having about five-
fold the rates in the lowest rate countries. The highest documented
rates are now in countries of Eastern Europe and the former USSR
and lowest rates are in the United States. In the last few decades,
most countries have experienced a decline in stroke rates. However,
such declines should not be taken for granted since they appear to
be levelling out, particularly in younger cohorts. Even within any
country, stroke rates vary by social class and geographic region. For
example, in Britain there are threefold regional variations with lowest
rates in the south and highest in the north, and there is a two- to
threefold gradient between persons in social class V and persons in
social class I.

Risk factors for stroke and implications for prevention

The large variations observed in stroke rates indicate the potential for
prevention. Raised blood pressure is the major known risk factor for
stroke in the population. Levels of systolic and diastolic pressure
both independently predict stroke. The risk increases steeply and
continuously with increasing blood pressure level with no threshold:
the higher the blood pressure, the higher the stroke risk over the

whole distribution of blood pressure, with relative risks increasing by nearly twofold for every 10 mmHg increase in diastolic blood pressure. In addition, numerous treatment trials of reduction of blood pressure have demonstrated reduction of stroke risk of about 35–40% for a 5–6 mmHg reduction in diastolic blood pressure; treatment of isolated systolic hypertension is also of benefit. In contrast, raised blood cholesterol, which is a powerful risk factor for coronary heart disease, is not consistently related to stroke. This is probably due to a positive association with ischaemic stroke and a negative association with haemorrhagic stroke. Nevertheless, trials of cholesterol reduction using statins have suggested benefits for stroke reduction. Many other factors have been implicated as predictive of stroke: these include raised fibrinogen, raised homocysteine and lower albumin levels, raised white cell count, chronic infection, poor respiratory function, diabetes and/or impaired glucose tolerance, and obesity. However, there is as yet no evidence from intervention trials that changes in levels of these risk factors will reduce stroke risk.

Many potentially modifiable lifestyle factors have also been implicated in stroke. These include cigarette smoking, physical activity, and a broad range of dietary factors. These have been directly linked with stroke risk in prospective studies, or have been demonstrated to influence stroke risk factors such as blood pressure. Of these, sodium has figured the most prominently, though its role is still controversial. On balance, the circumstantial evidence that sodium is important in influencing hypertension and stroke risk in populations is considerable. The magnitude of effect applied to the population has been estimated at about 10 mmHg blood pressure difference for every 100 mmol difference in sodium intake, or about 34% difference in stroke risk. Other dietary factors which have been related to blood pressure levels include potassium, magnesium, calcium, dietary fibre, omega-3 fatty acids, saturated fat, vitamin C, protein, and alcohol, but again the relationship with stroke is more uncertain. Dietary factors may have effects other than on blood pressure; for example, antioxidant vitamins are thought to protect against free radical damage affecting endothelial function or haemostasis, and folate may protect by influencing homocysteine levels. Many of the protective factors are found in fruit and vegetables and it is notable that several studies have reported a strong, protective effect of high fruit and vegetable intake on stroke; the magnitude of effect is considerable with an estimated 25–40% reduction in stroke risk for an increase of two to three servings of fruit or vegetables daily.

Conclusions

Stroke is a devastating but preventable condition. We already have ample evidence of effective interventions in high-risk groups such as treatment of hypertension and atrial fibrillation and carotid endartectomy for those with carotid stenosis. In Britain there have been substantial declines in stroke rates in the past few decades, but these declines appear to be levelling off, particularly in younger cohorts. While interventions in high-risk groups are still a priority, the ageing of the population poses a particular challenge for the future and we also need to identify effective preventive strategies for the whole population. Much evidence suggests that modifiable lifestyle factors may profoundly influence stroke risk in individuals and stroke rates in the community. Ongoing research is aimed at identifying and clarifying the role of existing and new interventions, particularly in groups such as women and older persons in whom there is a dearth of evidence. Meanwhile, current general health recommendations to increase fruit and vegetable intake to five servings a day, to increase physical activity, to reduce processed food intake (thus reducing sodium and saturated fat intake), and to reduce cigarette smoking are likely to be of benefit not just for stroke but for general health.

Further reading

Collins, R., Peto, R., MacMahon, S., Hebert, P., Fiebach, N. H., *et al.* (1990). Blood pressure, stroke, and coronary heart disease. Part 2. Short-term reductions in blood pressure: overview of randomised drug trials in their epidemiologic context. *Lancet*, **335**, 827–38.

Frost, C. D., Law, M. R., Wald, N. J. (1991). By how much does dietary salt reduction lower blood pressure. I: Analysis of observational data within populations. *Br. Med. J.*, **302**, 815–19.

Gillman, M. W., Cupples, A., Gagnon, D., Posner, B. M., Ellison, R. C., Castelli, W. P. (1995). Protective effect of fruits and vegetables on development of stroke in men. *J. Am. Med. Assoc.*, **273**, 1113–17.

Khaw, K. T. (1996). Epidemiology of stroke. *J. Neurol., Neurosurg., Psychiatry*, **61**, 333–8.

Prospective Studies Collaboration (1995). Cholesterol, diastolic blood pressure, and stroke: 13 000 strokes in 450 000 people in 45 prospective studies. *Lancet*, **346**, 1647–53.

4   Feasible methods of removal/reduction of risk factors

DR HELEN RODGERS

Senior Lecturer in Stroke Medicine
University of Newcastle upon Tyne

Although three-quarters of stroke patients are aged over 65 years, stroke is not an inevitable consequence of ageing but a disease which is potentially preventable at all ages. A number of risk factors have been identified which, if reduced by lifestyle changes or medical treatment, will potentially have a major impact on stroke incidence and mortality.

Large, well-conducted studies have demonstrated that treatments such as control of high blood pressure, the use of aspirin following a transient ischaemic attack (TIA) or stroke, carotid endarterectomy for symptomatic severe carotid stenosis, stopping smoking, and the use of warfarin in non-valvular atrial fibrillation can reduce the incidence of subsequent stroke. Despite clear evidence of benefit, recent research suggests that opportunities for prevention are being missed.

Successful stroke prevention requires an understanding of the prevalence of risk factors, individual risk, population attributable risk, patients' perceptions of risk, the effectiveness of approaches to risk factor reduction, and the effectiveness of implementation strategies. Research to date has focused on identifying and modifying risk factors but relatively little has been carried out to look at improving the implementation of effective lifestyle changes or medical treatments. At the present time stroke prevention is not optimal because the available knowledge is not being fully applied.

From an epidemiological perspective there are two approaches to stroke prevention: the high-risk strategy which targets individuals who are at the greatest risk of having a stroke, and the population approach which aims to reduce stroke risk factor levels for the population as a whole. For example, in terms of preventing stroke by reducing hypertension, the high-risk approach would involve good blood pressure control in patients who are known to be hypertensive and identification and treatment of hypertension in patients with other stroke risk factors. The population-based approach would involve encouraging the population as a whole to change their lifestyle in ways which would result in a reduction of blood pressure, e.g. exercise and dietary salt reduction.

In order to maximize opportunities for stroke prevention, a multidisciplinary intersectoral approach is needed, involving not only professionals and policy makers from health services but also education, the food industry, with valuable input from the public and charities such as The Stroke Association. The effectiveness of stroke prevention programmes depends not only on health professionals' knowledge and attitudes towards implementing effective treatments, but also on patients' views and perceptions of risk and benefits of behaviour modification or treatment, and further work is needed in both of these areas.

Hypertension is probably the most important modifiable risk factor for stroke. If blood pressure was adequately identified and treated in the UK, it has been estimated that this would result in a 38% reduction in stroke incidence. Although systematic reviews and evidence-based guidelines for the treatment of hypertension are available, the identification of people with high blood pressure and subsequent control remains poor, particularly in older people. Publishing hypertension guidelines alone does not lead to improved clinical practice. Current evidence suggests that the quality of care can be improved by computer packages, quality assurance, or education but their relationship with patient outcomes is not clear. In clinical practice, few patients seem to know their last blood pressure reading or what a normal blood pressure should be. There are enormous opportunities for health promotion, education, and to involve patients in self-monitoring.

The prevalence of atrial fibrillation (AF) rises with age and is 4.7% in people aged over 65 years. This group of patients has a significantly increased risk of stroke, particularly when other risk factors are present. Anticoagulation of these patients is a very effective means of stroke prevention, reducing the risk of subsequent stroke by 67%. Indeed, the benefit may be higher as this figure reflects the benefits on an 'intention to treat analysis'. However, anticoagulants are underused in these patients, particularly amongst the elderly who may be the most likely to benefit – only a quarter of those with AF, without contraindications to anticoagulation, are receiving this treatment. The benefits of anticoagulation in patients in reducing stroke risk depend upon the risks of warfarin, which in turn depends upon patient selection and levels of control. Clearly the NHS needs to look at ways of increasing levels of anticoagulation in patients with AF, and expansion of anticoagulant services will be needed. Half of all AF patients aged over 65 could be identified from GP prescribing records and opportunistic checking of the pulse rhythm in the surgery could identify a large proportion of the remainder. Available guidelines regarding anticoagulation for patients with AF are available in many health districts but are at times contradictory. Appropriate detection and treatment of this group of patients could prevent 3000–5000 strokes in the UK.

About 10% of stroke patients have a preceding transient ischaemic attack. The risk of stroke is greatest within the first few weeks of TIA. A number of hospitals have established neurovascular clinics for the rapid assessment and treatment of these patients but the direct and indirect effects of these clinics in terms of stroke prevention is not clear. Patients with TIA or ischaemic stroke benefit from antiplatelet agents, and hospital-based audits suggest that most receive these treatments. The National Sentinel Audit for Stroke 1998 found that 88% of patients with ischaemic stroke were prescribed aspirin. Carotid endarterectomy is extremely beneficial for patients with severe symptomatic carotid stenosis, but in our neurovascular clinic only 4% of patients with TIA fulfil these criteria. Therefore carotid endarterectomy, although very effective for individual patients, has little impact upon the incidence of stroke. Screening for carotid stenosis would not contribute significantly to stroke prevention.

There is a close response, reversible relationship of risk between cigarette smoking and stroke. Within five years of stopping smoking the risk returns to that of people who had never smoked. Nicotine replacement therapy nearly doubles cessation rates and has an additive effect to giving advice or more intensive support.

Although there is no clear relationship between stroke and serum cholesterol, recent evidence suggests that statins can reduce stroke incidence by 31% in patients with ischaemic heart disease. The benefits of lowering serum cholesterol in terms of stroke prevention in other groups of patients, particularly those with TIA or ischaemic stroke, is unclear.

Conclusion

At a population level, control of blood pressure, smoking cessation, and anticoagulation of patients with atrial fibrillation are the most important risk factors that need to be addressed if stroke incidence is to be significantly reduced in the UK. There is a need to ensure that current knowledge is implemented effectively, particularly in primary care where most patients with these risk factors will be identified, treated, and monitored.

Further reading

Ebrahim, S., Davey Smith, G. (1996). Health promotion effectiveness reviews. *Health promotion in older people for the prevention of coronary heart disease and stroke.* Health Education Authority, London.

Raw, M., McNeill, A., West, R. (1999). Smoking cessation: evidence-based recommendations for the health care system. *Br. Med. J.,* **318**, 182–5.

Sudlow, M., Thomson, R., Thwaites, B., Rodgers, H., Kenny, R. A. (1998). Prevalence of atrial fibrillation and eligibility for anticoagulants in the community. *Lancet,* **352**, 1167–71.

Warlow, C. P., Dennis, M. S., van Gijn, J., Hankey, G. J., Sandercock, P. A. G., Bamford, J. M., *et al.* (1996). *Stroke: A practical guide to management.* Blackwell Science, Oxford.

Wolf, P. A. (1998). Prevention of stroke. *Lancet,* **353** (Suppl. III), 15–8.

Section 2

Secondary prevention

5   Blood pressure (pre- and post-stroke hypertension)

PROFESSOR J. F. POTTER

Division of Medicine for the Elderly
The Glenfield Hospital, Leicester

In the UK there are still over 120 000 strokes per annum, of which 20% will be due to a recurrence. Primary stroke reduction must come from attacking the major risk factors, of which hypertension remains the number one treatable cause. Data from prospective observational studies have highlighted the strong association between blood pressure (BP) levels and stroke incidence for both cerebral haemorrhage and infarction, a 10 mmHg increase in diastolic BP being associated with an 80% increase in stroke risk.[1] However, the BP/stroke relation varies with age, the gradient being much steeper in younger than older subjects, and the attributable stroke risk due to hypertension decreases with age with <20% of strokes in the 65-year-old group being related to raised BP levels compared with 50% in the 45–54 year-old group. The type of hyper-tension also affects stroke risk, particularly in older age groups – isolated systolic hypertension has a greater relative risk than diastolic hyper-tension (3.2 compared to 2.1) when compared to normotensives. Although there has been much debate about a J-shaped relation-ship between BP and stroke, recent studies have shown this to be log linear for age groups up to 75+ years. However, the relation between BP and stroke in the 80+ year-old age group is nowhere near as clear and in fact some studies have shown an inverse relation.

Treatment of raised BP levels reduces primary stroke incidence by about 35% and this is true for both combined and isolated systolic hypertension.[2] Thiazide diuretics are a proven first-line therapy though recently, particularly in the isolated systolic hypertension treat-ment trials, initial therapy with dihydropyridine calcium channel blockers has been shown to be of benefit. However, it is important to appreciate that it is BP levels on treatment that are a much stronger predictor of stroke incidence than pre-treatment levels and it is therefore important not just to make the diagnosis but to make sure of adequate BP control. It is insufficient just to treat BP alone and other stroke risk factors such as smoking, diabetes mellitus, and atrial fibrillation should be sought and treated appropriately and a healthy lifestyle encouraged, i.e. reducing weight and excessive alcohol intake and increasing physical exercise.

Following acute stroke, BP levels are frequently elevated and have been shown to be an adverse prognostic indicator.[3] However, as yet, we do not know whether there are benefits in reducing BP in the acute post-stroke period and the majority of physicians tend to stop antihypertensive medication in the first few days post stroke. To date there have been no large randomized trials of BP modification in the acute phase and these are much needed. Currently there seems little evidence to suggest that pharmacologically altering BP acutely is of value, unless there are other pressing medical reasons, e.g. hypertensive encephalopathy for at least the first one to two weeks after cerebral infarction.

Almost 50% of stroke survivors will have elevated BP levels six months or more after the acute event. Although raised BP levels are a strong risk factor for primary stroke, the relation with stroke recurrence is nowhere near as clear. To date there have only been two randomized intervention studies of the treatment of hypertension post stroke and three further studies that have involved both normotensive and hypertensive transient ischaemic attack and stroke subjects. In hypertensives, non-fatal stroke recurrence was not significantly reduced by active treatment though combined fatal and non-fatal stroke events were reduced by 35%.[4,5] Taking all intervention studies including normotensives and hypertensives, fatal stroke recurrence was not reduced but total number of strokes were by 23% and all major cardiovascular events by one-fifth. There are current ongoing studies looking specifically at the treatment of BP in the post-acute period and these are awaited with interest.

Although it is clear that reducing BP levels is an effective primary preventative measure in reducing stroke incidence, many questions still remain unanswered. Is antihypertensive treatment of benefit in the very elderly or following stroke? When after stroke should antihypertensive medication be started, and at what level should treatment be instigated, and what are the best antihypertensive agents to use in these patients? Hopefully some of these questions will be answered by ongoing studies, but, until then, in the acute and post-stroke periods at least we will have to rely on our clinical judgement with regard to the use of antihypertensive medication.

References

1. Prospective Studies Collaboration (1995). Cholesterol, diastolic blood pressure, and stroke: 13 000 strokes in 450 000 people in 45 prospective cohorts. *Lancet*, **346**, 1647–53.
2. Gueyffier, F., Froment, A., Gouton, M. (1996). New meta-analysis of treatment trials of hypertension: improving the estimate of therapeutic benefit. *J. Hum. Hypertens.*, **10**, 1–8.
3. Robinson, T., Waddington, A., Ward-Close, S., Taub, N., Potter, J. (1997). The predictive role of 24-hour compared to casual blood pressure levels on outcome following acute stroke. *Cerebrovasc. Dis.*, **7**, 264–72.
4. Carter, B. A. (1970). Hypotensive therapy in stroke survivors. *Lancet*, **19**, 485–9.
5. Hypertension–Stroke Cooperative Study Group (1974). Effect of antihypertensive treatment on stroke recurrence. *J. Am. Med. Assoc.*, **229**, 409–18.

6   Anticoagulants in stroke prevention

Dr G. S. VENABLES

Consultant in Neurology
Royal Hallamshire Hospital, Sheffield

In 80% of cases, stroke is the result of the consequences of arterial occlusion from fibrin, platelets, red cells, cholesterol, or fragments of atheroma. Anticoagulants (AC) reduce the effects of arterial occlusion elsewhere in the body and therefore might reduce the consequences of occlusion within the arteries supplying the brain. Unfortunately, these agents also cause both extra- and intracranial haemorrhage, the consequences of which are rarely trivial and are often fatal. Their use, therefore, must be based on an assessment of not only their theoretical benefit but also knowledge of the balance of benefit and risk in real-life clinical practice.

Acute stroke intervention

Evidence concerning the use of AC in acute stroke is based on more than 16 randomized controlled trials in over 20 000 patients. In some trials patients have received new low-molecular-weight heparins, but in most, standard heparins were used in doses varying from low, subcutaneously to high, intravenously. CT was not mandatory prior to treatment in all trials. Treatment took place up to seven days after onset. Efficacy measures varied with early trials examining the effect on deep vein thrombosis, one trial looked at death within 14 days and death or dependency at six months, while others used different functional outcome measures deemed to be 'favourable'.

In patients with atrial fibrillation there is nothing to be gained from starting treatment within the first seven days after acute stroke and treatment can be deferred until the deficit has recovered in patients with minor stroke, and after 1–2 weeks in those with a more substantial deficit. There is, therefore, a large cohort of heterogenous patients treated in a variety of ways to examine whether a policy of early treatment with an anticoagulant might have any effect on death or later dependency.

A systematic review of this policy[1] (level 1a evidence) suggests that there is no benefit in treating people with anticoagulants in the first week after stroke. Of those treated with heparin, 11.7% died or had non-fatal recurrent stroke in hospital compared with 12.1% of those not so treated. After six months there was no difference in the proportion dead or dependent and the number damaged from intracranial haemorrhage offset any benefit in the use of heparin. One trial using low-molecular-weight heparin suggested benefit and further trials are awaited. There is level 3 evidence of efficacy in preventing deterioration in special circumstances, e.g. thrombosing basilar artery.

Secondary prevention

Patients with cardiac disease may be at high risk of subsequent stroke and there have been a number of small studies, many done before the advent of CT, that may have included patients with primary intracranial haemorrhage. A recent systematic review[2] showed an excess of intracranial haemorrhage that may have offset any benefit, in terms of preventing ischaemic stroke. One recent trial has disclosed results of comparing a policy of stroke prevention with anticoagulants with a policy of prevention with aspirin. This included patients with recent (<6 months) transient ischaemic attack (TIA), and with minor or major non-disabling stroke who were not in atrial fibrillation and in whom there was <70% carotid stenosis, and showed that treatment with AC was associated with significant hazard terms of fatal and non-fatal intracranial haemorrhage.[3] Certain subgroups were at greater risk, including older patients, hypertensive patients, and those with extensive subcortical white matter disease. This study used a target INR 3.0–4.0. Two further studies are awaited, but the evidence would suggest that at the present time there is no benefit, and some hazard, to the policy of treatment with AC and antiplatelet drugs are the treatment of choice.

Patients with mechanical cardiac disease are at particular risk of embolic stroke and it has been customary to treat those with mechanical, e.g. valvular, heart disease with anticoagulants. On the basis of the published evidence a level C recommendation can be made about the use of AC in rheumatic valve disease, mitral valve prolapse, mitral annular calcification, aortic valve disease, cardiomyopathy, mechanical heart valves other than for second generation valves (level B), and bioprosthetic valves. There is rather more evidence to support the addition of aspirin in patients who continue to have emboli despite adequate anticoagulation. In acute myocardial infarction, heparin should be reserved for those at special risk, including those in atrial fibrillation.

There is level 1a evidence for the efficacy of AC in the prevention of first-ever stroke in patients with atrial fibrillation[4,5] with a 68% (95% CI 50–79%) reduction in risk of stroke, 68% (95% CI 39–83%) reduction in risk of disabling stroke, and 33% (95% CI 9–51%) reduction in risk of death in treated patients. Older patients with additional risk factors should be offered AC, younger patients without other risk factors need only be offered treatment with antiplatelet drugs. Those with previous cerebral thromboembolic events, hypertension, diabetes, or heart failure are at highest risk and have most to gain from the use of long-term anticoagulants.

References

1. Counsell, C., Sandercock, P. (1997). Efficacy and safety of anticoagulant therapy in patients with acute presumed ischaemic stroke: a systematic review of the randomized trials comparing anticoagulants with controls. The Cochrane Collaboration. Issue 1. Update Software, Oxford.
2. Liu, M., Counsell, C., Sandercock, P. (1997). *Anticoagulation versus no anticoagulation following non-embolic stroke or transient ischaemic attack*. The Cochrane Collaboration. Issue 1. Update Software, Oxford.
3. The SPIRIT Trial Investigators (1997). Secondary Prevention of Recurrent Ischaemia Trial. *Ann. Neurol.*, **42**, 857–65.
4. Atrial Fibrillation Investigators (1994). Risk factors for stroke and efficacy of antithrombotic therapy in atrial fibrillation. Analysis of pooled data from five randomized controlled trials. *Arch. Intern. Med.*, **154**, 449–57.
5. European Atrial Fibrillation Trial Study Group (1993). Secondary prevention in non-rheumatic atrial fibrillation after transient ischaemic attack or minor stroke. *Lancet*, **342**, 1255–62.

7 Antiplatelet therapy for the secondary prevention of stroke or transient ischaemic attack

DR JOHN BAMFORD

Consultant Neurologist and Cerebrovascular Physician
St James' University Hospital, Leeds

Introduction

The use of antiplatelet therapy for patients with stroke or transient ischaemic attack (TIA) represents a significant therapeutic success although one has to be realistic about the likely magnitude of benefit from any single therapy in a condition where there are many different causative mechanisms. Furthermore, as is often the case, a piece of scientific information both informs clinical practice but also raises further questions. Thus, the fact that questions are still being asked about what constitutes optimal antiplatelet therapy should not detract from the importance of the evidence that we currently have.

Background

The logic for using antiplatelet therapy for secondary stroke prevention is compelling. About 85% of all strokes and TIAs are caused by cerebral ischaemia and, amongst these patients, between 7 and 12% will have a further stroke each year.[1] We also know that there is greater death and disability after a recurrent stroke than after a first stroke or TIA.[2,3] Recurrent symptoms commonly occur because of blood clot (thrombus) building up and occluding either large or small arteries to the brain (thrombosis) or because of thrombus being carried to, and blocking, the brain (embolism). The platelets in the blood are known to have a critical role in the formation of thrombus and platelet thrombi have been seen passing through the retinal circulation in patients having ocular TIA. Therefore it seems logical that strategies which reduce the tendency of platelets to form thrombus might reduce the rates of recurrent stroke.

The aspirin story

As far back as the 5th century Hippocrates was using the extract of willow bark to relieve the pain of childbirth. In 1763, a clergyman called Edmund Stone reported to the Royal Society about the effects of chewing willow bark in 50 of his parishioners. The active ingredient was salicylic acid but this was highly irritant to the stomach. The reaction between salicylic acid and acetyl chloride which produced acetyl salicylic acid was patented by Bayer in 1899 and the compound was called aspirin. The mechanism of action of aspirin was finally identified in 1971 by Professor John Vane.

It was soon recognized that patients who were taking aspirin would bleed for up to three times longer than patients who were not taking the drug. The earliest reports of the use of aspirin in patients with vascular disease came from an American physician who reported his impression that patients taking the drug survived longer than equivalent patients who were not taking the drug. Other such anecdotal reports followed during the 1960s – one needs to remember that this was before the advent of the randomized, controlled clinical trial as the gold standard of treatment studies. However, the landmark publication by Professor Fields and colleagues[4] in 1977 of their trial of the use of aspirin in patients with TIA set the scene for two decades of intense clinical trial activity which ends with it no longer being ethical to have a placebo group in any secondary stroke prevention trial, such is the overwhelming acceptance of the efficacy of aspirin in this clinical setting.[5]

Scratch the surface of this consensus, however, and one will find continuing debate about a number of important clinical issues. Perhaps the most contentious is what dose of aspirin should be used. For simplicity, consider aspirin dosages to be either high (>900 mg/day), medium (about 300 mg/day), or low (<100 mg/day). Early trials all used high doses whereas more recent trials have used lower and lower doses. The only really robust way to compare the efficacy of two drugs or two doses of the same drug is to study them in the same randomized trial primarily so that one can be sure that the patients receiving the treatments are as similar as possible (so-called direct comparison). Trying to compare the outcome in patients in different trials (so-called indirect comparison) is fraught with potential biases and it is often when this type of analysis is used that there is both scientific disagreement and clinician confusion. There are only two trials that provide direct comparison data: the UKTIA trial compared high (1200 mg) and medium (300 mg) doses[6] whilst the Dutch TIA trial compared medium (283 mg) and low (30 mg) doses.[7] In neither case was there a statistically significant difference in outcome between the two doses. Indirect comparison using meta-analysis supports the view that there is not likely to be a significant difference in efficacy between dosages but there never has been, nor is there ever likely to be, a trial that directly compares high and low doses. There is, however, a considerable reduction in risk of side-effects (predominantly gastrointestinal) with the lower doses and, therefore, most European doctors recommend doses of 300 mg/day or lower, but some North American experts continue to recommend 1200 mg/day.

Taking aspirin after stroke or TIA reduces the risk of a further serious vascular event by between 10 and 20% – a useful benefit from a cheap and relatively safe drug. Nevertheless, there are several pathways of platelet activation which are not blocked by aspirin. Newer drugs, such as dipyridamole and clopidogrel, which block different pathways of platelet activation to aspirin have been shown to reduce the risk of serious vascular events after a stroke or TIA. The findings of the ESPS2 trial, in which the combination of dipyridamole and aspirin was more efficacious than either agent alone, lends support to the biologically plausible hypothesis that blocking more than one pathway of platelet activation may result in greater protection against serious vascular events.[8,9] It is always going to be more difficult to show with certainty that one efficacious drug (or combination of drugs) confers greater protection than another, particularly when using indirect comparisons, and this is probably the main reason for the ongoing debate about the place of these newer agents in everyday clinical practice. Inevitably, the notoriously murky subject of 'cost-effectiveness' gets raised and there may well be a place for trying to identify those patients with stroke or TIA who are at highest risk of a subsequent major vascular event.

Just over the horizon there are potentially even more efficacious antiplatelet drugs (the GIIb/IIIa antagonists) which are just beginning to enter phase III clinical trials. In the meantime, probably the single most beneficial thing that doctors can do is to ensure that, unless there are specific contraindications, all their patients who have had an ischaemic stroke or TIA are taking antiplatelet therapy.

References

1. Bamford, J. M., Sandercock, P. A. G., Dennis, M. S., Burn, J., Warlow, C. P. (1990). A prospective study of acute cerebrovascular

disease in the community: The Oxfordshire Community Stroke Project 1981–1986. *J. Neurosurg. Psychiat.*, **53**, 16–22.

2. Dennis, M., Burn, J., Bamford, J., Sandercock, P., Warlow, C. (1993). The Oxfordshire Community Stroke Project: Long-term survival after first-ever stroke. *Stroke*, **24**, 796–800.

3. Burn, J., Dennis, M., Bamford, J., Sandercock, P., Warlow, C. (1994). Stroke recurrence in a population-based cohort. The Oxfordshire Community Stroke Project. *Stroke*, **25**, 333–7.

4. Fields, W. S., Lemak, N. A., Frankowski, R. F., Hardy, R. J. (1977). Controlled trial of aspirin in cerebral ischemia. *Stroke*, **8**, 301–14.

5. Antiplatelet Trialists' Collaboration (1994). Collaborative overview of randomised trials of antiplatelet therapy. 1. Prevention of death, myocardial infarction, and stroke by prolonged antiplatelet therapy in various categories of patients. *Br. Med. J.*, **308**, 81–106.

6. The UK TIA Study Group (1991). The United Kingdom Transient Ischaemic Attack (UK TIA) Aspirin Trial: final results. *J. Neurol., Neurosurg., Psychiat.*, **54**, 1044–54.

7. The Dutch TIA Study Group (1991). A comparison of two doses of aspirin (30 mg vs. 283 mg a day) in patients after a transient ischemic attack or minor ischemic stroke. *N. Engl. J. Med.*, **325**, 1261–6.

8. Diener, H., Cunha, L., Forbes, C., Sivenius, J., Smets, P., Lowenthal, A. (1996). European Stroke Prevention Study 2. Dipyrimadole and acetylsalicylic acid in the secondary prevention of stroke. *J. Neurol. Sci.*, **143**, 1–13.

9. CAPRIE Steering Committee (1996). A randomised blinded trial of clopidogrel versus aspirin in patients at risk of ischaemic events (CAPRIE). *Lancet*, **348**, 1329–39.

Section 3

Management of stroke

Coordinated stroke care

DR PETER LANGHORNE

Senior Lecturer in Geriatric Medicine
Academic Section of Geriatric Medicine, University of Glasgow

Introduction

Coordinated care for stroke patients in hospital is an old concept which has received increased attention over the last decade.[1] For many years there has been controversy about whether the recovery of stroke patients in hospital could be improved if their care was provided in a coordinated, organized manner; an approach that has been termed 'stroke unit' care. In 1989, a review of rehabilitation strategies concluded that 'convincing evidence concerning the therapeutic usefulness of stroke rehabilitation does not yet exist'.[2] This article explores the evidence supporting coordinated stroke unit care and its implications in terms of (a) how this information may have influenced current stroke care, and (b) the direction of future research.

We should first consider what we mean by coordinated stroke unit care. The definition can be broad ('any system of in-patient care which aimed to improve the organization of stroke patient care'[1]), but has been further developed in the light of the available trials (see below) such that it has come to mean 'coordinated multidisciplinary team care for stroke patients in hospital'.

What are the potential benefits of coordinated stroke unit care?

We can address this using the systematic review of 20 clinical trials which compared coordinated care provided by a stroke unit (stroke ward or stroke team) with conventional care which was usually provided in the general medical ward.[3] This indicated that patients who were managed in a coordinated stroke unit setting were more likely to survive, return home, and regain physical independence after their stroke. For every 100 patients receiving stroke unit care, three additional patients would survive, three would avoid institutional care, and six additional patients would return home – the majority of whom would be independent in daily activities. These benefits were seen in both male and female patients, young and elderly, and in those with mild or severe strokes. The benefits were observed with stroke units which either admitted patients immediately after stroke or accepted later referrals for rehabilitation. Benefits were also apparent in units which managed stroke patients together with other disabling illnesses as well as those which focused only on stroke patients. These findings have recently gained independent support from a major national survey of stroke care in Sweden[4] which found that patients managed in a stroke unit were more likely to survive and return home.

Having established that coordinated stroke unit care provides a more effective way of managing stroke patients, we need to explore the resource implications of such an approach. In most Western countries the main determinants of the cost of acute stroke care relate closely to the length of stay in hospital because the major health care costs are due to nursing care and hospital overheads.[5] This is certainly true in countries such as the UK where a relatively non-intensive approach to stroke care is provided. The longer-term costs of stroke care are largely attributable to the care of dependent individuals in hospitals or nursing homes.[6] Therefore it follows that coordinated stroke unit care should have advantages over conventional care if it reduces long-term disability without increasing the cost of an episode of in-patient care or the length of stay in a hospital or institution. The data from randomized trials suggest that the number of individuals surviving without major disabilities is increased without resulting in any systematic increase in the length of hospital stay.[3] The net increase in the cost of an episode of care is likely to be modest and certainly outweighed by the potential benefits of coordinated stroke unit care.[1]

What are the lessons from the stroke unit trials?

The stroke unit trials have demonstrated that a complex package of coordinated care in hospital can result in important improvements in stroke patient recovery. We therefore need to establish what lessons we can learn and, in particular, which measures we should introduce into current practice and which should be subject to further research.

A descriptive analysis of the stroke unit trials[1] identified four areas of practice which were significantly different between the stroke unit and conventional care settings.

1. *Coordinated multidisciplinary team care provided by staff with a specialist interest in stroke care.* The most characteristic feature of coordinated stroke unit care was the presence of a multidisciplinary team (nursing, medical, physiotherapy, occupational therapy, speech and language therapy, social work) of staff who had a specialist interest in stroke care and met on a weekly basis to provide a coordinated package of care for stroke patients. Nursing practices were closely coordinated with this multidisciplinary process and carers were encouraged to become involved at an early stage. This aspect of care was universally present in stroke unit settings and almost always absent from conventional care settings, and so it could be considered a defining characteristic of stroke unit care. This finding has allowed the definition of a basic service specification for both the commissioning and auditing of stroke services. Both the Stroke Association Survey of Stroke Services and the Scottish Stroke Services Audit have used this definition of care. This has also encouraged a range of research activities exploring the nature of coordinated multidisciplinary team care. For example, research at the University of Newcastle has sought to measure the knowledge, skills, and attitudes of nurses working with stroke patients. Research in London is exploring the similarities and differences between units dedicated to stroke patients and other more generic multidisciplinary settings. Finally, groups such as the British Association of Stroke Physicians are beginning to define the training requirements of staff working with stroke patients.

2. *Programmes of education and training in stroke care.* The stroke unit services in the clinical trials routinely provided information to patients and carers about stroke disease and also had programmes of education and training for staff. This observation has encouraged the further specification of coordinated stroke services as incorporating programmes of education and training. The role of information provision in stroke rehabilitation has recently become the subject of randomized trials and a planned systematic review.

3. *Intensity of rehabilitation.* The stroke units studied did not always provide a more intensive programme of physiotherapy or occupational therapy, although in a minority of cases this did occur. However, it did appear that the net amount of rehabilitation activity

was increased within the stroke unit settings,[1] partly through the extended role of rehabilitation nurses. This observation should encourage research in two areas: (i) the impact of a more extended rehabilitation nursing role to provide a greater amount of rehabilitation activity throughout the patient's day; and (ii) randomized trials of the intensity of rehabilitation input to identify if the additional cost of increasing this results in improved patient outcomes. At least four recent randomized trials and two systematic reviews have been carried out.

4. *Comprehensive care.*   Patients who were managed in coordinated stroke unit settings were more likely to have an assessment by a physiotherapist or occupational therapist, and this was more likely to occur at an earlier stage. A very active, early mobilization programme was a distinctive characteristic feature in those units which accepted patients acutely. This raises the question of whether we should be carrying out randomized trials of early mobilization – although many practitioners now believe that this is good practice and would not be appropriate for a clinical trial. The early medical management is another area for future attention. It is notable that several effective units had detailed policies to improve early care such as the provision of intravenous saline infusions, routine use of paracetamol to lower body temperature, a low threshold for using antibiotics, and careful checking for the need of oxygen or insulin. Although these individual components are not supported by randomized trials, some acute stroke units are already adopting this type of policy.

It is interesting to note a recent pilot study from Newcastle which demonstrated that early monitoring and intervention reduced the number of patients whose condition deteriorated over the first few days.[7]

Conclusions

The last decade has seen a major change in attitudes with most clinicians now accepting that coordinated stroke unit care is an effective package of care. The uncertainties now are how best to implement such care. Hopefully the next decade will help us identify reliable and widely applicable systems of care which can be applied throughout the UK.

References

1. Langhorne, P., Dennis, M. (1998). Stroke units: an evidence-based approach. BMJ Books, London.
2. Dobkin, B. H. (1989). Focused stroke rehabilitation programs do not improve outcome. *Arch. Neurol.*, **46**, 701–3.
3. Stroke Unit Trialists' Collaboration (1999). *Organized in-patient (stroke unit) care for stroke.* Issue 1. Update Software, Oxford.
4. Stegmayr, B., for the Steering Committee of 'RIKS-Stroke' (1998). 'RIKS-Stroke': the Swedish national hospital registry for quality assessment of acute stroke care. *Cerebrovasc. Dis.*, **8**, 1–103.
5. Warlow, C. P., Dennis, M. S., van Gijn, J., *et al.* (1996). *Stroke: A practical guide to management.* Blackwell Science, Oxford.
6. Evers, S. M. A. A., Engel, G. L., Ament, A. J. H. A. (1997). Cost of stroke in the Netherlands from a societal perspective. *Stroke*, **28**, 1375–81.
7. Davis, M., Hollymann, C., McGiven, M., Chambers, I., Egbuji, J., Barer, D. (1998). *Physiological monitoring in acute stroke.* British Geriatrics Society conference proceedings.

9   Acute treatment and coordinated care

PROFESSOR PHILIP BATH

Professor of Stroke Medicine
Nottingham City Hospital

Stroke is a clinical syndrome and follows brain ischaemia (85% of patients), primary intracerebral haemorrhage (PICH, 10%), or subarachnoid haemorrhage (5%). Acute ischaemic stroke results from a cascade of vascular and neuronal events initiated by thromboembolic occlusion of arteries and reduced regional cerebral blood flow.[1] The resulting ischaemia leads to neuronal dysfunction and, ultimately, cell death. Most haemorrhagic strokes follow rupture of micro-aneurysms or are secondary to amyloid angiopathy. Either way, bleeding induces pressure-related local ischaemia. Both ischaemia and haemorrhage manifest themselves as focal neurological disturbance typically presenting with one or more of weakness, sensory loss, altered vision, cortical deficits such as dysphasia, or posterior fossa signs such as ataxia, depending on which arterial territory is involved. The long-term sequelae include death in one-third of patients, and dependency in another third.

Acute stroke is a medical emergency and patients with stroke symptoms should be reviewed at hospital without delay. Ideally, general practitioners should not intervene in acute stroke since seeing the patient at home introduces a significant delay in arrival at hospital. Patients should be assessed in the emergency room for the clinical diagnosis of stroke. Emergency resuscitation with oxygen, fluids, or metabolic control may be necessary and swallowing function assessed. The principal investigation is brain CT scanning which will exclude other intracranial pathologies mimicking stroke, distinguish between ischaemic stroke and PICH, and help determine prognosis.

Patients should be admitted to an acute stroke unit for multidisciplinary care involving acute treatment, further investigation, prevention of complications, early rehabilitation, and secondary prevention. Such units facilitate clinical care and research although their effect on outcome is unclear. Once patients are medically stable and investigations are complete, those needing continuing rehabilitation should be transferred to a stroke rehabilitation unit; such dedicated units are now known to reduce death, improve functional outcome, and reduce hospital length of stay.[2]

Considerable effort has gone into developing specific treatments for ischaemic stroke, focusing on reperfusion and neuroprotective strategies. The very large International Stroke Trial (IST) found that aspirin reduces the risk of early reinfarction and late death and disability.[3] Although the effect of aspirin on outcome is small, its clinical utility is wide and its cost is low. A potentially more potent treatment strategy involves intravenous thrombolysis. Unfortunately, conflicting trial results and the significant risk of intracranial haemorrhage have prevented its early introduction.[4,5] A large trial involving 2500+ patients is now required to resolve whether thrombolysis can be given safely and effectively. Other promising vascular approaches include intra-arterial thrombolysis and defibrinogenation. In contrast, unfractionated heparin appears to be of no benefit in ischaemic stroke.[3]

Neuroprotection is based on the hypothesis that ischaemic neurones can be protected during periods of reduced regional cerebral blood flow. A number of different neuroprotective protocols have been tested, including inhibiting glutamate release, antagonizing glutamate or polyamine receptors, blocking N-methyl-D-aspartate (NMDA) ion channels, blocking voltage-dependent calcium channels, scavenging free radicals, and inhibiting phagocyte activity through blocking endothelial adhesion molecules.

Unfortunately, none of these approaches has been successful. A large trial of intravenous magnesium (Intravenous Magnesium Efficacy Study, IMAGES), a NMDA ion channel blocker and cerebral vasodilator, is currently underway in acute stroke. Radical neuroprotective approaches for the management of cerebral oedema and intracranial hypertension have been promulgated recently, specifically the induction of moderate hypothermia (31 °C to 33 °C) or surgical hemicraniectomy, although no randomized controlled trials have tested these to date.

Considerably less attention has been paid to the treatment of PICH than ischaemic stroke. Although unproven, actively bleeding posterior fossa strokes should be surgically evacuated or shunted to prevent brainstem compression and hydrocephalus. Whether surgery has a role in the management of supratentorial intracerebral haemorrhage is currently uncertain and is being studied in the Surgical Treatment of Intracranial Haemorrhage (STICH) trial. Since areas of haemorrhage are typically surrounded by ischaemia, it is also possible that neuroprotectants might be effective – no efficacy studies have addressed this hypothesis to date.

The acute management of associated medical problems, in particular dysphagia, hypertension, hyperglycaemia, and pyrexia, remains unclear although each is independently associated with a worse prognosis. Feeding approaches in dysphagia are being studied in the large Feed Or Ordinary Diet (FOOD) trial. An efficacy study of the management of hyperglycaemia has started recently (Glucose Insulin in Stroke Trial, GIST). Definitive studies are now needed to assess how best to manage blood pressure and temperature during the acute phase of stroke. In the meantime, stroke physicians should probably attempt to normalize blood glucose and temperature; blood pressure is best left untreated in most patients since active lowering may worsen outcome, at least with some antihypertensive drug classes.

Deep vein thrombosis and pulmonary embolism complicate stroke. Although practised widely, the use of compression leg stockings to prevent thromboembolism has not been proven in stroke in spite of them being effective in other high-risk groups of patients. However, rehydration and early mobilization (and aspirin in ischaemic stroke) should all reduce this risk.

The UK is a major player in the design and running of large acute stroke trials, witness IST in the past, and FOOD, GIST, IMAGES, and STICH now. Additionally, the rise of evidence-based practice makes it is increasingly important that adequate UK sources of funding are available to support future academic phase III randomized controlled trials and the undertaking of systematic reviews in acute stroke. However, such trials must be larger and use up-to-date trial design and outcome measures as compared with their forebears.

References

1. Bath, P. M. W. (1997). The medical management of stroke. *Int. J. Clin. Pract.*, **51**, 504–10.
2. Stroke Unit Trialists' Collaboration (1997). *Specialist multidisciplinary team (stroke unit) care for stroke in-patients*. In: Stroke Module of the Cochrane Database of Systematic Reviews [updated 4 March 1997] (ed. C. Warlow, J. van Gijn, P. Sandercock). Available in The Cochrane Library (database on disk and CD-ROM). The Cochrane Collaboration. Update Software, Oxford.
3. International Stroke Trial Collaborative Group (1997). The International Stroke Trial (IST): a randomised trial of aspirin, subcutaneous heparin, both, or neither among 19 435 patients with acute ischaemic stroke. *Lancet*, **349**, 1569–81.

4. The National Institute of Neurological Disorders and Stroke rt-PA Stroke Study Group (1995). Tissue plasminogen activator for acute stroke. *N. Engl. J. Med.*, **333**, 1581–7.
5. Hacke, W., Markku, K., Fieschi, C., *et al.* (1998). Randomised, double-blind, placebo-controlled trial of thrombolytic therapy with intravenous alteplase in acute ischaemic stroke (ECASS 11). *Lancet*, **352**, 1245–51.

10 Management of depression and related disorders after stroke

DR A. HOUSE

Consultant and Senior Lecturer in Liaison Psychiatry
Department of Psychiatry, University of Leeds

Depression, like other mood disorders, has a number of components. There is the experienced emotion – depression, unhappiness, or dysphoria; cognition such as hopelessness, helplessness, suicidal thinking, ideas of worthlessness, or guilt behaviours including crying, withdrawal from social life, or self-harm; and physical symptoms such as loss of appetite or libido.

One way to assess mood is to aggregate these elements into a symptom score. This is the approach adopted by self-report questionnaires such as the Beck Depression Inventory. Its rationale is that the more symptoms somebody has, the more likely they are to be suffering from a clinically important condition. A second approach is to concentrate on those symptoms believed to have diagnostic significance. This is the rationale behind self-report scales such as the Hospital Anxiety and Depression Scale and the use of diagnostic syndromes (such as major depressive disorder) described in DSM IV and ICD 10. The main advantage of the syndromal approach is that it allows some prediction of response to treatment. For example, the major depressive syndrome is frequently used as an indication for antidepressant medication. The third approach is to disaggregate and concentrate on individual items such as apathy, hopelessness, or tearfulness. Such individual symptoms may be important in predicting outcome but it is an area that has been little researched in stroke.

Bearing in mind this uncertainty about the appropriate definition of depression, what treatments are available?

Treatments for establishing depression

Antidepressants are widely used – some 20–30% of survivors are prescribed one in the first year after stroke. Under the circumstances it is surprising that there is little evidence about their effectiveness.

There is only one published study which describes a conventional randomized controlled trial (RCT) in which an antidepressant was compared to placebo: mood was measured by a standardized method, more than 50 patients were randomized, and an intention-to-treat analysis was conducted.[1] Even in this study the numbers were relatively small, the sample was recruited at widely different times after stroke, and follow-up was only for six weeks. Therefore we do not know the costs and benefits of antidepressant medication after stroke. Also, there are no published trials of psychological treatment for depression after stroke.

The result is that in choosing a treatment we must rely on generalizing from evidence in other areas. There is reasonable evidence that depression in the physically ill responds to antidepressant drugs,[2] but the costs are unclear and there is no evidence about which drug to use. There is evidence that psychological treatments work in other settings but none in relation to stroke – where one might have reservations because of the associated communication and cognitive problems.

Preventing the development of depression

If treatments for established depression are disappointing, should we concentrate more on prevention?

There are (perhaps surprisingly) a number of studies which have examined the role of antidepressant medication in preventing the development of depression or in improving physical outcome after stroke. They suffer from the methodological problems referred to above. Their results have been essentially negative, and again they have raised the concern of unacceptably high rates of adverse effects in the stroke population.

The most substantial body of published research describes the effect of psychosocial intervention aimed at preventing depression after stroke. In a recent review[3] these trials were categorized into four main groups:

(1) *education* – involves the provision of written or oral information about stroke and its after-effects. It differs from information provision by virtue of involving an interactive session between the educator and the recipient of the information;
(2) *leisure therapy* – a specific form of occupational therapy which aims to enhance mood and self-esteem by encouraging active

involvement in activities which subjects have themselves defined as rewarding or enjoyable;

(3) *stroke support workers* – the rationale for stroke support workers is not always made explicit but there are two likely components. One is the bolstering of the social network by provision (at least temporarily) of additional members. The other is the additional opportunity to have stroke-related problems identified and dealt with by the existing services;

(4) *counselling* – there are many theoretical models underlying talking therapies, but the common theme is that there is the opportunity to talk to an independent person as a means of exploring dilemmas and identifying solutions to them.

These approaches are popular with patients and carers, and they improve satisfaction with services. However, they do not seem effective in preventing depressive disorders. Nonetheless, we should not be too hasty in dismissing them. The quality of the trials in which they have been evaluated is poor, and it may be that an important effect is being missed. Brief and non-intensive therapies are unlikely to be effective unless they are delivered by a therapist experienced in the field who has had a specific training and supervision in delivery of the therapy.

A research agenda for the future

Clarifying the role of drugs

We do not know the full range of indications for psychotropic medication after stroke, or the costs and benefits of medication. We do not even know the costs and benefits of antidepressive medication for major depressive disorder after stroke, despite the substantial rates of prescribing of these drugs. These questions could be answered by a conventional RCT, planned and conducted to currently accepted quality standards.

What are the other indications for psychotropic medication after stroke? For example, do antidepressant drugs hold any benefit for patients with depressive symptoms but who do not meet the diagnostic criteria for the major depressive syndrome? Other symptoms for which antidepressants are prescribed include apathy and emotional lability.[4] The symptoms seem to respond in some cases but we do not know whether it is solely those people who have an associated depressive disorder who benefit.

Finally there is the question of the role of psychostimulants such as metylphenidate and dexamphetamine either in depression or apathy.

Developing and evaluating specific psychological therapies

Future research into psychosocial intervention after stroke should of course be designed to the highest quality standards and should at the same time take account of three deficits which are relatively specific to this area.

First, the intervention should be based on a theory about the causes of depression associated with severe physical illness. This may not be as straightforward as it seems. For example, helping people with their problems after stroke might seem a common-sense way of improving their mood. But everybody has some problems after stroke and not everybody gets depressed, so it must be some other characteristic which defines those who do. An effective intervention might not be to work at removing problems but might involve teaching the patient problem-solving skills – so-called problem-solving therapy[5] – or challenging maladaptive styles of thinking as in cognitive therapy.

Second, the therapy being evaluated should be delivered in a clearly described and standardized way. This means not just that its theory should be enunciated but that the content of each session should be described. In practice this nearly always means that it should be manual based.

Third, the therapy should be delivered by a therapist with the appropriate level of clinical experience and adequate training and supervision.

Conclusion

There are now effective treatments for depression with a sound theoretical and empirical justification. Our main task in the next few years is to commission and undertake good quality research which will establish the place of such treatments in stroke rehabilitation.

References

1. Andersen, G., Vestergaard, K., Lauritzen, L. (1994). Effective treatment of post-stroke depression with the selective serotonin reuptake inhibitor Citalopram. *Stroke*, 25, 1099–104.
2. Gill, D., Hatcher, S. (1999). A systematic review of the treatment of depression with antidepressant drugs in patients who also have a

physical illness [Cochrane review]. The Cochrane Library. Issue 1. Update Software, Oxford.

3. Knapp, P., Young, J., House, A., Forster, A. (In press.) A review of non-drug strategies to resolve psychosocial difficulties after stroke age and ageing. *Age and Ageing*.

4. Brown, K., Sloan, R., Pentlan, B. (1998). Fluoxetine as a treatment for post-stroke emotionalism. *Acta Psych. Scandinav.*, 98, 455–8.

5. Hawton, K., Kirk, J. (1997). Problem solving. In: *Cognitive–behaviour therapy for psychiatric patients – a practical guide* (2nd edn). Oxford University Press, Oxford.

Section 4

Surgical/medical treatment

11   Intracranial surgical | procedures for stroke

PROFESSOR A. DAVID MENDELOW

Consultant in Neurosurgery
Newcastle General Hospital, University of Newcastle

Introduction

As with occlusive stroke, surgical treatment can be divided into *preventative* and *therapeutic*. Preventative surgery may be primary or secondary, as is the case for carotid endarterectomy in asymptomatic and symptomatic carotid stenosis. So with intracranial procedures, treatment of asymptomatic aneurysms can be regarded as primary and treatment of ruptured aneurysms as secondary. The same applies to surgical or interventional radiological treatment of arteriovenous malformations (AVMs). The evacuation of an intracerebral haemorrhage (ICH) would always be regarded as secondary. Similarly, decompressive craniotomy for brain swelling following carotid occlusion would also be regarded as secondary.

A major part of the work of any neurosurgical unit is the primary surgical treatment of conditions that cause haemorrhagic stroke. The secondary treatment of complications includes the removal of haematomas and control of elevated intracranial pressure (ICP) by medical and surgical means.

Preventative surgery

Aneurysms

Primary clipping or coiling of unruptured aneurysms is undertaken when the risk of rupture is high and where the patient has a reasonable life expectancy. The recent Mayo Clinic study[1] has indicated that small aneurysms (<10 mm) on the anterior circulation have a low risk of bleeding; by contrast, a large basilar aneurysm carries a much higher risk and intervention is required. Whether craniotomy with clipping or coiling is undertaken depends upon the risks in each case, and these depend upon the anatomy of the aneurysm and the track record of the surgeon or radiologist.

Arteriovenous malformations

The risk of haemorrhage from an unruptured AVM was also documented from the Mayo Clinic[2] and is 3% per year. In about 15% of cases the lesion can be obliterated by angiographic embolization with glue. In small (<2 cm) AVMs, stereoradiosurgery will occlude 90% of lesions. Larger AVMs require a combination of embolization followed by craniotomy. The risks of this multimodality treatment have been summarized by Spetzler and Martin.[3]

Occlusive stroke

Treatment of intracranial arterial stenosis or occlusion by angioplasty or extracranial to intracranial arterial (ECIC) bypass is not of proven benefit at present although clinical trials to evaluate these procedures are being considered. New techniques of angioplasty using stents and new forms of bypass using the radial artery or the saphenous vein are being developed.

Surgical treatment of established haemorrhage or infarction

Aneurysms

A comparison between craniotomy with clipping and angiographic coiling of ruptured aneurysms is currently being undertaken (ISAT trial).

Arteriovenous malformations

It is unusual to treat these lesions acutely unless they are associated with an ICH that requires surgical removal. Under these circumstances, the AVM may be removed at the time of craniotomy.

Intracerebral haemorrhage

In some patients with large, superficial haematomas where there is secondary deterioration in the level of consciousness or the neurological deficit, surgery is indicated. In the majority of patients an expectant policy is adopted. However, in many patients the surgeon is uncertain about the need for evacuation and a meta-analysis has indicated that neither surgical nor conservative treatment has proven benefit.[4] A prospective randomized controlled trial (Surgical Treatment of Intracranial Haemorrhage, STICH) is under way, funded by The Stroke Association and the Medical Research Council. More than 130 patients have been randomized to date. It is anticipated that 1000 patients would be needed to show a 10% benefit from surgery.

Intraventricular haemorrhage

When this is associated with hydrocephalus, ventricular drainage is indicated. The prognosis from intraventricular haemorrhage is poor but drainage may be life-saving in some cases.

Cerebral infarction

In patients with brain swelling from established infarction, good results have been claimed for decompressive craniotomy.[5] However, prospective randomized controlled trials have not been undertaken in these circumstances and, until completed, the successful reports must be regarded as anecdotal. Similarly, intensive care management with ICP monitoring and ventilation is an interesting but as yet unproven treatment.

References

1. Investigators, The International Study of Unruptured Intracranial Aneurysms (1998). Unruptured intracranial aneurysms – risk of rupture and risks of surgical interventions. *N. Engl. J. Med.*, **339**, 1725.
2. Brown, R. D., Wiebers, D. O., Forbes, G. S. (1990). Unruptured intracranial aneurysms and arteriovenous malformations: frequency of intracranial haemorrhage and relationship of lesions. *J. Neurosurg.*, **73**, 859–63.
3. Spetzler, R. F., Martin, N. A. (1986). A proposed grading system for arteriovenous malformations. *J. Neurosurg.*, **65**, 476–83.
4. Hankey, G. J., Hon, C. (1997). Intracerebral haemorrhage. *Stroke*, **28**, 2126–32.
5. Delashaw, J. B., Broaddus, W. C., Kassell, N. F. (1990). Treatment of right hemisphere cerebral infarction by hemicraniectomy. *Stroke*, **21**, 874–81.

12 Carotid endarterectomy

ALISON HALLIDAY

Consultant in Vascular Surgery
Epsom General Hospital and St George's Hospital, London

History

Over a century ago, in 1856, Savory recorded his examination of a young woman who had right hemiplegia and a history of left monocular symptoms; he found at post-mortem that the left internal carotid artery was occluded.[1] The association of cerebral symptoms with carotid artery narrowing was further strengthened in 1914 when Ramsey Hunt declared that no post-mortem examination of cerebral infarction could be considered complete unless the neck arteries were also examined.[2] Not long after, in 1927, Moniz performed the first carotid angiogram, and for the first time it became possible to diagnose carotid occlusion whilst the patient was still alive.[3]

Formal surgical intervention was not proposed until Miller Fisher in 1951 suggested 'it is even conceivable that some day vascular surgery will find a way to bypass the occluded portion of the artery during the period of ominous fleeting symptoms'.[4] The first recorded report of this was made by Eastcott, *et al.* in 1954 – a woman complaining of frequent transient ischaemic attacks (TIAs) had successful resection of a portion of tightly stenosed carotid artery.[5]

Carotid surgery: the fall and rise

The popularity of removing atheromatous carotid arterial narrowing (endarterectomy) has waned since 1985. By then it had become the fourth commonest operation in the United States, although Britain lagged (and still does) far behind. At that time over 100 000 operations were being undertaken yearly in the US, and the process of auditing results was far from optimal. However, it was clear that there were wide differences in indications for, and results of, carotid endarterectomy, with reported stroke rates caused by operation varying between 2 and over 20%.

In 1991, two large, prospective randomized controlled trials were reported simultaneously, identifying who should (and who should not) definitely have this operation. The North American Symptomatic Carotid Endarterectomy Trial (NASCET)[6] and European Carotid Surgery Trial (ECST)[7] examined several thousand symptomatic (mild stroke or TIA) patients allocated to surgery (and appropriate medical treatment) versus medical treatment alone. Surgery was beneficial in patients with narrowing of 70–99%, but hazardous in those with under 30% stenosis. The intermediate group, with the exception of some with 60–69% stenosis, did not do better with operation.

This should have ensured that fewer, but more appropriate, operations were subsequently undertaken, but further trials have now suggested that some patients *without* symptoms may also be best treated by operation. To understand why this is possible, it is necessary to consider the likely operative mortality and morbidity. For previously symptomatic patients, around 5% will have a stroke or die as a result of surgery. This risk is less if they had a TIA rather than mild stroke. If patients with tight stenosis but no symptoms are operated on, prophylactically about 3% will suffer these complications. Without operation, stroke risk also rises with more severe presenting symptoms making the balance of risk dependent on the results of surgery.

There is now good evidence that prophylactic endarterectomy can halve the risk of stroke in patients with 60–99% stenosis, but half of a low stroke risk (around 2% per year) is a small benefit. Carotid endarterectomy is expensive (£3000 in the UK), and asymptomatic carotid stenosis is common. If all the people in the UK who had this were operated on, only 4% of all first-in-a-lifetime strokes would be prevented, and the bill for the NHS would be enormous. Attitudes in the US differ from here and endarterectomy rates have now soared since the Asymptomatic Carotid Atherosclerosis Study (ACAS) reported that prophylactic operation prevented stroke.[8] It is likely that a balance may be struck in future when the results of the final trial in prophylactic surgery are known. The Asymptomatic Carotid Surgery Trial (ACST)[9] is funded by The Stroke Association and the UK Medical Research Council and is likely to report around 2003 on whether a high-risk group can be identified who might have greater benefit from preventive operation than that suggested by ACAS.

Carotid endarterectomy: the operative procedure and hazards

Operation may be carried out under general or local anaesthetic. The patient is prepared and an incision made in the skin along the medial border of the sternomastoid muscle. The carotid sheath containing carotid and jugular vessels and vagus nerve is exposed. After giving heparin, the internal, external, and common carotid arteries are prepared (taking care to avoid damaging the XIIth [hypoglossal] and IXth [glossopharyngeal] nerves nearby) and clamped. A plastic heparinized shunt may be used to carry blood from common to internal arteries whilst the atheromatous narrowing is removed. Once the diseased portion has been excised, the artery is washed out with heparinized saline solution and carefully closed so as not to cause any significant narrowing. A fine suction drain is placed and the wound closed in appropriate layers. The patient is awakened and returned to the recovery room, high dependency, or intensive care unit. Discharge is usually possible within three or four days.

The main operative hazard is stroke. The patient may awake with a neurological deficit, or it can develop, usually within the first six hours. Stroke can be caused by the dissection when preparing the artery, allowing friable material from the atheroma to be carried into the (usually) middle cerebral artery, leading to infarction of cerebral cortex. After endarterectomy, the surface of the artery is highly thrombogenic, and stroke can develop when internal carotid artery flow is reduced or occluded by clot.

Measures undertaken to avoid stroke include the intraoperative measurement of middle cerebral arterial pressure by transcranial doppler (ultrasound), use of shunts, measurement of flow in the operated carotid vessels with on-table duplex doppler, or on-table angiography. Meticulous anaesthetic and surgical care are necessary, and the operation has the reputation of being the most demanding in the vascular surgeon's repertoire – conceptually simple, but potentially disastrous, with results immediately apparent to patient and carers. Successful surgery saves stroke and reduces the risk of further stroke on the operated side to around 0.5% per annum.

References

1. Savory, W. S. (1856). Case of a young woman in whom the main arteries of both upper extremities and of the left side of the neck were throughout completely obliterated. *Med. Chir. Trans. Lond.*, **39**, 205–19.
2. Hunt, J. R. (1914). The role of the carotid arteries in the causation of vascular lesions of the brain, with remarks on certain special features of the symptomatology. *Am. J. Med. Sci.*, **147**, 704–13.
3. Moniz, E. (1927). L'encephalographie arterielle: son importance dans la localisation des tumeurs cerebrales. *Rev. Neurol.* (Paris), **2**, 72–90.

4. Fisher, M. (1954). Occlusion of the carotid arteries. *Arch. Neurol. Psychiat.*, **2**, 187–204.
5. Eastcott, H. H. G., Pickering, G. W., Rob, C. (1954). Reconstruction of internal carotid artery in a patient with intermittent attacks of hemiplegia. *Lancet*, **2**, 994–6.
6. North American Symptomatic Carotid Endarterectomy Trial Collaborators (1991). Beneficial effects of carotid endarterectomy in symptomatic patients with high-grade carotid stenosis. *N. Engl. J. Med.*, **325**, 445–53.
7. European Carotid Surgery Trialists' Collaborative Group (1991). MRC European Carotid Surgery Trial: Interim results for patients with severe (70–99%) or with mild (0–29%) carotid stenosis. *Lancet*, **337**, 1235–43.
8. Executive Committee for the Asymptomatic Carotid Atherosclerosis Study (1995). Endarterectomy for asymptomatic carotid artery stenosis. *J. Am. Med. Assoc.*, **273**, 1421–8.
9. Halliday, A. W. (1994). The Asymptomatic Carotid Surgery Trial (ACST): rationale and design. *Eur. J. Vas. Surg.*, **8**, 703–10.

13

Angioplasty

PROFESSOR MARTIN M. BROWN

Professor of Stroke Medicine
Institute of Neurology, London

Narrowing of the carotid arteries in the neck (carotid stenosis) secondary to atherosclerosis is an important cause of stroke. Previous clinical trials, including the European Carotid Surgery Trial (ECST),[1] have shown that surgical removal of severe carotid stenosis is beneficial in preventing subsequent stroke after warning symptoms of transient ischaemic attack (TIA) or non-disabling stroke.

However, surgery has disadvantages, including a risk of stroke at the time of the procedure and the risks of complications caused by the incision in the neck. These include injury to cranial nerves, haematoma, wound infection, and a scar. Most surgeons prefer to perform carotid surgery under a general anaesthetic, which has its own risks.

In contrast, treating carotid stenosis by percutaneous transluminal balloon angioplasty (PTA) avoids the risks of the incision in the neck and is usually conducted under local anaesthetic. Good anatomical results can be obtained, with no more discomfort to the patient than occurs during routine carotid angiography. However, PTA risks stroke at the time of the procedure. The need to insert a balloon catheter through the stenosis may cause cerebral embolism and inflation of the balloon may cause injury to the wall (carotid dissection).

The results of earlier series of carotid angioplasty were encouraging, with reported risks at the time of the procedure similar to that of carotid surgery.[2] However, the risks and benefits in comparison to surgical treatment were uncertain. Therefore an international, multi-centre randomized trial was conducted to compare the safety and benefits of angioplasty with surgery, known as the Carotid and Vertebral Artery Transluminal Angioplasty Study (CAVATAS).[3] A total of 504 patients with carotid stenosis were randomized at 24 centres in the United Kingdom, Europe, Australia, and North America between surgery and angioplasty. Surgery was carried out using conventional carotid endarterectomy. Angioplasty was carried out using balloon catheters.

In the later stages of the study, some patients were also treated with stenting, a procedure in which a wire mesh is expanded inside the stenosis, usually after balloon dilation, to hold open the artery. Follow-up in CAVATAS was carried out by independent neurologists. The primary analysis of safety data showed no difference by intention to treat in the risks of stroke or death occurring during, or within 30 days of, either treatment. However, the 30-day morbidity rate of stroke or death in both arms was 10%.

However, carotid angioplasty avoided cranial nerve injury and had a significantly lower rate of haematoma, requiring surgery or prolonging hospital stay. The analysis of follow-up data showed that angioplasty and surgery were equally effective at preventing subsequent stroke after treatment and there was no difference in the rate of stroke during follow-up. However, restenosis was significantly more common in the patients treated by angioplasty on ultrasound examination at 12 months after treatment. Restenosis rarely caused symptoms during follow-up.

In conclusion, angioplasty is a hopeful alternative to surgery for carotid stenosis but further clinical trials are required before the procedure can be introduced widely. It is hoped that the use of stents in all cases, together with protection filters to prevent emboli during stent insertion, will improve the safety of the procedure. Therefore a new trial is starting, known as the International Carotid Stenting Study, in which primary carotid stenting will be compared with carotid surgery in suitable symptomatic patients with severe carotid stenosis. It is hoped that the trial will confirm that carotid angioplasty and stenting provide a less invasive alternative to surgery for the prevention of stroke.

References

1. European Carotid Surgery Trialists' Collaboration Group (1998). Randomised trial of endarterectomy for recently symptomatic carotid stenosis: final results of the MRC European Carotid Surgery Trial. *Lancet*, **351**(9113), 1379–87.
2. Brown, M. M. (1998). Angioplasty for stroke prevention. In: *Cerebrovascular disease: pathophysiology, diagnosis, and management* (ed. L. Ginsberg, Bogousslavsky), pp. 1931–44. Blackwell Science, Oxford.
3. The CAVATAS investigators. Results of the Carotid and Vertebral Artery Transluminal Angioplasty Study (CAVATAS). (In preparation for submission to *Lancet*.)

14   Evidence for invasive intervention: where do we go from here?

PROFESSOR CHARLES P. WARLOW

Professor of Medical Neurology
Department of Clinical Neurosciences, University of Edinburgh

Most 'invasive' interventions are surgical. Exceptions include angio-plasty, embolization of material to occlude abnormal vessels, and even, perhaps, nasogastric tubes. For present purposes, I will confine myself to surgical operations but the same principles apply to other invasive interventions. Whether a patient is referred to a surgeon from a physician, which is usually the case, or directly, there are five questions to be addressed before recommending surgery.

What is normal practice?

Increasingly, guidelines are defining normal practice but their formulation depends on good data, preferably from randomized controlled trials (RCTs) and meta-analyses. If the data do not exist, or are poor, then practice will vary, whatever the guidelines say. Indeed, without good data the guidelines are likely to hedge and use unhelpful phrases such as 'the treatment should be considered' (as though we need reminding!).

How good is the surgeon?

Politicians and patients think this is an easy question to answer, largely by looking at outcomes after surgery. Implicitly this conjures up 'league tables'. This approach is both naive and potentially damaging to the surgeons at the bottom of the table. With very few exceptions, a surgeon will not be doing enough of a particular operation to have results which are statistically stable enough not to be influenced by chance. And even when they are stable, the outcomes have to be adjusted for case-mix, an all but impossible task even with well-validated prognostic models, which are themselves thin on the ground. Of course there is also the problem of bias – a surgeon with what appears to be poor results is likely to obscure them (and so is a physician, but this is harder to detect, which is why most league tables are all about surgery and not about drugs).

How good is the surgery?

The answer comes most reliably from RCTs. In the stroke area there is very good information about carotid endarterectomy, and there will be good information eventually about carotid angioplasty and surgery for intracerebral haematoma. Without RCTs we are relying on not much more than guesswork, whim, prejudice, and what happened to the last case.

Is the patient prepared to take a risk?

Inevitably, any invasive intervention carries a risk, as indeed does any effective drug. The unique thing about surgery death is, however, that so often the risk is very obvious and taken early (perioperative death, etc.) and the benefit comes later (a longer life). So it is crucially important that an individual patient understands this trade-off and is prepared to take it. To do so, he or she needs to know what the risk of surgery is for them personally, and what the outlook would be without surgery. But RCTs only give 'on average' answers to these questions, and we need to go further. After all, although patients with severe symptomatic carotid stenosis have a high risk of stroke (maybe 30%), they do not all have a stroke and for the 70% who do not, surgery is unnecessary.

Will this individual patient benefit from surgery?

This is where the cutting edge of research now lies, particularly for carotid endarterectomy where we know what the 'on average' effects are for recently symptomatic patients with severe carotid stenosis. With difficulty, we and others are trying to define reliable ways of picking out the smallish numbers of patients who *will* have a stroke from the large number who *might*, and then to offer safe surgery to just these patients. This sort of approach will never be perfect but at least it should reduce the 'numbers needed to treat' for one patient to avoid a stroke from about nine now, to maybe three or four in the future.

And what of the future? The grey area of uncertainty

As well as examining the data we do have from RCTs, usually in individual patient data meta-analyses, it is obvious that more RCTs are needed, both of existing treatments and of new treatments. For surgical interventions this has always been regarded as more difficult than the evaluation of drugs. In fact it is not, and in many ways it is easier (there is no problem with long-term compliance, or what dose to use, for example). Also, the 'generalizability' of the results of surgical trials is no more of a problem than it is for the non-randomized surgical series (issues of quality of surgery, the type of patient operated on, etc.).

In essence the problem boils down to the resistance of so many surgeons to the concept of randomization, and ethics. This can be solved by exploiting what is known as 'the grey area of uncertainty'. In real life there are patients for whom one is sure, for whatever reason good or bad, that a treatment should be used, and so one uses it and it would be unethical not to. There are other patients for whom the treatment appears to be definitely not useful, and it would be unethical to use it. Both categories of patient could not possibly be asked to enter an RCT. It would be ethically unsustainable and bad science because for those patients the science is solved in the mind of the doctor; the treatment works for the first category, not for the second. But there is always a middle group for whom one is genuinely uncertain whether to use a treatment or not – the 'grey area'. In this group the best science flows from randomizing the patients to the treatment or not, to find out for that sort of patient whether, on average, the treatment works. This is also the best ethics because the alternative is to recommend, or not, a treatment when one is not sure whether that is the most effective option. If the patients knew this then they would surely agree, but so often in normal practice they are far from fully informed about the uncertainties (with the best of intentions, often to protect them from being troubled by those very uncertainties).

Furthermore, patients in RCTs are not just contributing knowledge for future patients, they are themselves gaining – they have the potential advantage of a treatment which has been carefully thought about and peer reviewed, or the potential advantage of avoiding some unforeseen adverse effect of that treatment; their records will be carefully taken and kept for a matter of years; they are likely to be treated by experts in their disease who are educating all the other doctors involved in the trial; any ancillary treatments are likely to be appropriate in an atmosphere of collaboration amongst experts; they are likely to be followed up very carefully; and any risk is likely to be monitored very carefully, often by independent people. It is no wonder that even the 'no treatment' (control) patients in RCTs so often do better than expected.

The future will see treatments being better assessed and with guidelines based on more evidence. And, with any luck, we will be able to focus the treatments more accurately on those who really need them.

Further reading

European Carotid Surgery Trialists' Collaborative Group (1998). Randomised trial of endarterectomy for recently symptomatic carotid stenosis: final results of the MRC European Carotid Surgery Trial (ECST). *Lancet*, **351**, 1379–87.

Lindley, R. I., Warlow, C. P. Why and how should trials be conducted? In: A. Zeman, L. Emanuel (ed.) *Ethical dilemmas in neurology*. W. B. Saunders, London. (In press.)

Rothwell, P. M., Warlow, C. P. on behalf of the European Carotid Surgery Trialists' Collaborative Group (1999). Analysis of treatment effects in individual patients: prediction of benefit from carotid endarterectomy. *Lancet*, **353**, 1325.

Warlow, C. (1994). The design of controlled clinical trials. In: *Oxford textbook of surgery* (ed. P. J. Morris, R. A. Malt), pp. 2723–31. Oxford University Press, Oxford.

Warlow, C. P., Dennis, M., van Gijn, J., Hankey, G., Bamford, J., Sandercock, P., *et al.* (1996). *Stroke: A practical guide to management*. Blackwell Scientific, Oxford.

Section 5

Imaging

15   CT and MRI scanning in stroke

DR D. J. THOMAS

Consultant in Neurology
St Mary's Hospital, London

Introduction

Clinical assessment of a 'stroke patient' is very effective at localizing where the problem has occurred in the brain or spinal cord. However, it does not permit an accurate assessment of the nature of the stroke. Until 25 years ago the fundamental separation between the two main possibilities, namely a thrombosis leading to brain infarction or a cerebral haemorrhage, was not reliable. The acute medical treatment for these two conditions can be quite different so it is important to distinguish between them. It was the invention of computerized axial tomography scanning (initially called EMI scanning, then CAT, and now CT) by Sir Godfrey Hounsfield that permitted a quantum leap in diagnostic precision.

CT Scanning

CT brain scanning is very effective at identifying an intracranial haemorrhage almost immediately after the event. A haemorrhage shows as a bright white abnormality against a grey background. Not only can CT scanning show haemorrhages within the brain but it can also reveal subarachnoid haemorrhages and post-traumatic subdural and extradural haematomas. CT scanning was initially confined to neurosurgical centres, but over the last 20 years it has become widely available and most district general hospitals will have a scanner. Many more stroke patients can now be scanned than ever before. Lives can often be saved and neurological handicap dramatically reduced by such rapid detection and surgical treatment of these haemorrhages.

CT scanning can also identify infarcts but not quite so dramatically as haemorrhages. An infarct shows up as a grey area different from the normal surrounding brain. Sometimes the infarct may be difficult to see to the untrained eye. This may be because the infarct is small or because it is very recent so it has hardly had time to change much from normal.

There is currently great enthusiasm for clot-busting (thrombolytic) therapy in acute ischaemic (thrombotic) stroke. Before using such treatment we have to know that the patient has not had a haemorrhage and that the CT brain scan does not already show signs of an established infarct. (Sometimes the early signs of an infarct can be very subtle.) In both these situations clot-busting would be likely to cause a haemorrhage and make matters worse.

MRI

Magnetic resonance imaging (MRI) has some advantages over CT and has started to become more widely available over the last 10 years. Many stroke patients seen now have an MRI instead of a CT.

MRI is more sensitive than CT at showing cerebral infarction. It is more efficient at revealing fine brain structures and small ischaemic events are detected five times as easily on MRI as on CT. Newer imaging techniques with MRI, particularly diffusion-weighted imaging, are also more sensitive than CT at detecting very early cerebral thrombosis and fresh cerebral infarcts. So in centres where this technique is readily available, it is now the method of choice for early investigation of acute stroke.

MRI spectroscopy also permits some pathophysiological information to be obtained. This allows an assessment of the metabolic problems in and around a stroke and may be helpful in predicting the extent of the recovery.

MRI is also preferable to CT in assessing patients attending vascular clinics with transient ischaemic attacks (TIAs), or those with memory or other intellectual problems. It is now appreciated that TIA symptoms are a poor guide to disease activity. Patients presenting with a single TIA may have numerous ischaemic lesions on scanning. MRI can give very clear signs of the number, type, and distribution of these vascular lesions. It permits detection of silent infarcts in parts of the brain that are not obviously symptomatic. Preventative treatment can be monitored and new 'clinically silent' events can be spotted and therapy modified accordingly.

Angiography

Both CT scanning and MRI permit imaging of the intracerebral arteries and of the major feeding arteries in the neck. No injection of 'dyes' is required. No risk is involved. This information can be very helpful in assessing the cause of a stroke and in advising appropriate therapies. For example, thrombolytic therapy may be helpful if there is a fresh embolus lodged at the origin of the middle cerebral artery, while it is unlikely to be helpful if there is an occlusion of the internal carotid artery.

Present position

As a minimum, most patients presenting with a sudden stroke should have at least a CT scan of the brain to help refine the diagnosis and to guide targeted management. Where available, an MRI scan is in many instances preferable.

In special units, the 'state-of-the-art' advice is that patients should be admitted within two hours. They should then be assessed immediately with MRI brain scanning, including using diffusion-weighted imaging techniques to detect established infarcts. MR angiography can be obtained at the same time. Suitable patients can then proceed to thrombolytic therapy, where indicated, within three hours of the onset of the stroke.

Further reading

Sutton, D., *et al.* (1998). MRI spectroscopy: MR angiography: spiral CT angiography. In: *Textbook of radiology and imaging, Vol. 1* (6th edn) (ed. D. Sutton, *et al.*). Churchill Livingstone, London.

Warlow, C. P., Dennis, M. S., van Gijn, J., Hankey, G. J., Sandercock, P. A. G., Bamford, J. M., *et al.* (1996). *Stroke: A practical guide to management*. Blackwell Science, Oxford.

Welch, K. M. A., Caplan, L. R., Reis, D. J., Siesjo, B. K., Weir, B. (1997). *Primer on cerebrovascular diseases*. Academic Press, San Diego.

16   Ultrasound and transcranial Doppler

DR HUGH S. MARKUS

Reader in Neurology
Guy's, King's, and St Thomas' School of Medicine and
Institute of Psychiatry, London

Ultrasound is widely used as a simple, relatively cheap, and non-invasive method of imaging the extracerebral and intracerebral circulation. Using frequencies of the order of 5–7 MHz, it is possible to obtain both high-resolution B-mode images of the carotid arteries and Doppler information on blood flow velocity. This combination is usually referred to as duplex ultrasound. The skull attenuates, or absorbs, much ultrasound and, therefore, a lower-frequency ultrasound (2 MHz) has to be used for transcranial Doppler ultrasound. This results in images of much lower resolution and, therefore, the structural information that can be obtained is limited. However, useful information on blood flow velocity in the intracerebral vessels can be obtained.

Carotid ultrasound is widely used as a first-line screening method to detect carotid stenosis and identify patients who may be suitable for carotid endarterectomy. Stenoses can be detected both by a high-velocity jet through the narrowed lumen and the presence of atheromatous plaque on B-mode imaging. The technique is reliable if careful quality control is applied, and it is now used by some centres as the sole technique to identify patients for carotid endarterectomy.

Because of its non-invasive nature, carotid ultrasound is ideal for population studies. The high-resolution B-mode images can demonstrate early changes of atherosclerosis in the carotid arteries. Both increased intima-media thickness and the presence of plaques have been used as an index of the extent of atherosclerosis, and appear to be independent predictors of cardiovascular risk.[1] This technique may be useful in predicting risk in individual patients, and has also been widely used in determining the role of a number of novel risk factors in the pathogenesis of carotid atherosclerosis.

Transcranial Doppler ultrasound can be used to identify intracranial stenoses in vessels such as the middle cerebral artery; these are again identified by the presence of a high-velocity jet. This technique is widely used in some countries both in patients with acute stroke and also to look for vasospasm following subarachnoid haemorrhage. The technique can be used to identify children with sickle cell disease who have intracranial stenoses and are at particular risk of stroke. Recently it has been demonstrated in a large randomized study that stroke risk in these children can be markedly reduced by exchange transfusions, and transcranial Doppler remains the simplest technique by which such at-risk individuals can be identified.[2]

Using commercially available head straps, it is easy to hold the ultrasound transducer in place for prolonged periods, making transcranial Doppler ideally suited to monitor changes in cerebral blood flow velocity over time. For this reason it is widely used during interventional procedures, particularly carotid endarterectomy. It gives an index of cerebral perfusion and alerts the surgeon to potential problems such as shunt kinking. It is also used by many surgeons to identify which patients require shunting during the operation.

The high temporal resolution of the technique is also utilized in developing methods of studying cerebral autoregulation. This is the mechanism by which cerebral blood flow is maintained during changes in blood pressure. It plays a vital role in protection against brain ischaemia, but appears to be disturbed in diseases such as hypertension and brain injury. In the past it has been difficult to estimate, requiring complex measurements of cerebral blood flow in combination with drugs given to alter blood pressure. The increase in cerebral blood flow velocity in response to carbon dioxide, a potent cerebral vasodilator, has been used for many years as an indicator of the haemodynamic effect of a carotid stenosis or occlusion. It gives an indirect assessment of cerebral autoregulation, and of the effectiveness of collateral supply. Impaired carbon dioxide reactivity ipsilateral to a carotid occlusion identifies a group of patients at high risk of future stroke and transient ischaemic attack (TIA).[3] Recently it has been possible to determine cerebral autoregulation directly using transcranial Doppler. In a technique developed by Aaslid and colleagues, cuffs are inflated around the thighs and then suddenly deflated, resulting in a sudden small drop in blood pressure.[4] Following this, blood pressure slowly rises, but blood flow to the brain returns to normal much more rapidly, indicating the presence of cerebral autoregulation. By comparing the rate of rise of cerebral blood flow velocity measured by transcranial Doppler with the rate of rise of blood pressure, an estimate of cerebral autoregulation can be obtained. Using this technique it has been demonstrated that impaired cerebral autoregulation may occur in head injury and carotid stenosis.[5]

Recently there has been considerable interest in the use of transcranial Doppler to detect cerebral emboli. It was only in 1990 that it was appreciated that circulating cerebral emboli can be detected using Doppler ultrasound.[6] They reflect and scatter more of the ultrasound beam than the surrounding red blood cells and, therefore, appear as short-duration, high-intensity signals in the Doppler spectrum. They are accompanied by a characteristic clicking or chirping sound. The technique has been validated in a variety of models and asymptomatic embolization has been demonstrated in the cerebral circulation in patients with a number of at-risk states, including carotid stenosis and atrial fibrillation.[7] In certain situations, such as carotid stenosis and post-carotid endarterectomy, the presence of emboli appears to predict future stroke risk. This technique has a number of exciting applications. It may allow detection of patients at high risk of stroke for appropriate pharmacological or surgical treatment. For example, it may identify patients with asymptomatic carotid stenosis who would particularly benefit from carotid endarterectomy. It may also provide a technique by which new antiplatelet drugs can be evaluated. Current evaluation of such drugs requires very large clinical trials. Using asymptomatic embolic signals as a surrogate endpoint, and because they are very much more frequent than TIAs and strokes, the effectiveness of novel therapies can be screened in much smaller numbers of patients.

The low-frequency ultrasound required to allow transmission through the skull has limited the use of transcranial Doppler in studying the structure of the brain. More recently, an increasing number of transcranial duplex machines have become available which allow imaging of the intracerebral circulation. On the whole, the spatial resolution of these is poor but some useful information can be obtained. Their application may be improved by the use of ultrasound contrast agents.[8] These are composed of very small micro-bubbles which increase the amount of ultrasound reflected back from the blood vessels, and therefore the intensity of the signal. They may also be useful in the 10–20% of patients in whom transcranial Doppler signals cannot be obtained due to a lack of adequate ultrasound transmission through the skull. These agents are currently being evaluated in a number of clinical studies.

References

1. Bots, M. L., Hoes, A. W., Koudstaal, P. J., Hofman, A., Grobbee, D. E. (1997). Common carotid intima-media thickness and risk of stroke

and myocardial infarction: The Rotterdam Study. *Circulation*, **96**, 1432–7.
2. Adams, R. J., McKie, V. C., Hsu, L., Files, B., Vichinsky, E., Pegelow, C., *et al.* (1998). Prevention of a first stroke by transfusions in children with sickle cell anemia and abnormal results on transcranial Doppler ultrasonography. *N. Engl. J. Med.*, **339**(1), 5–11.
3. Kleiser, B., Widder, B. (1992). Course of carotid artery occlusions with impaired carbon dioxide reactivity. *Stroke*, **23**, 171–4.
4. Newell, D. W., Aaslid, R., Lam, A. M., Mayberg, T. S., Winn, R. (1994). Comparison of flow and velocity during dynamic autoregulation testing in humans. *Stroke*, **25**, 793–7.
5. White, R. P., Markus, H. S. (1997). Non-invasive determination of impaired cerebral autoregulation in carotid artery stenosis. *Stroke*, **28**, 1340–4.
6. Spencer, M. P., Thomas, G. I., Nicholls, S. C., Sauvage, L. R. (1990). Detection of middle cerebral artery emboli during carotid endarterectomy using transcranial Doppler ultrasonography. *Stroke*, **21**, 415–23.
7. Markus, H. S., Harrison, M. J. (1995). Microembolic signal detection using ultrasound. *Stroke*, **26**, 1517.
8. Postert, T., Federiein, J., Przuntek, H., Buttner, T. (1997). Insufficient and absent acoustic temporal bone window: potential and limitations of transcranial, contrast-enhanced, color-coded sonography and contrast-enhanced, power-based sonography. *Ultrasound Med. Biol.*, **23**(6), 857–62.

17 The future of stroke imaging

PROFESSOR P. M. MATTHEWS

Consultant in Neurology
Centre for Functional Magnetic Resonance
Imaging of the Brain, Dept. of Clinical Neurology
University of Oxford

Stroke remains a major medical problem. It has been identified as a major target for future development of neurological care. Current primary imaging goals are to define stroke pathology, to establish prognosis as early as possible, and to develop approaches for a sensitive imaging of the evolution of disease pathology in order to assess the efficacy of interventions rapidly. The importance of the latter goal will increase dramatically as new targets for pharmacological intervention are identified in the 'post-genome' era.

Magnetic resonance imaging (MRI) has become a critical tool in stroke imaging. Because of its flexibility and broad diffusion across medical centres, it is likely to become the major tool for both acute and chronic stroke monitoring. Magnetic resonance imaging on current systems can be used to provide quantitative information on brain pathology. Some highly specific information on changes in the biochemistry of tissues related to ischaemia is available, allowing monitoring of all aspects of pathological evolution in molecular detail. Finally, new approaches based on functional magnetic resonance imaging (FMRI) have allowed aspects of the neural system's reorganization associated with brain injury to be defined. Quantitative measures of this reorganization ultimately may be useful as indices of outcome with new pharmaceutical interventions or rehabilitation procedures.

Optimal acute stroke management demands early and accurate diagnosis. Experiments conducted on animals and later extended to man have defined clearly that there is a complex series of changes in water mobility that occurs in areas of necrotic tissue. Diffusion-weighted MRI imaging provides a measure of these changes in relative water diffusion.[1] Within two to three hours of the onset of severe ischaemia, the diffusion of water molecules within affected tissue decreases significantly. This appears to be due to mobility changes for smaller molecules in the cytoplasm, as well as the redistribution of water between the extracellular and intercellular spaces. Ischaemic tissue necrosis also leads to loss of diffusion anisotropy, reflecting the loss of the normal-oriented facilitation of diffusion along directions of axoplasmic flow in areas of white matter change. Over several days (generally 10–14) there is a progressive increase in the diffusion coefficient. After a 'pseudo-normalization' when the diffusion coefficient becomes equivalent to that of a normal parenchyma, the diffusion coefficient increases until it is higher than in normal tissue. Increased water diffusion is also associated with the long-term cystic changes in an infarct. Thus, in addition to providing a highly sensitive index of early change in ischaemic lesions, the relative ADC can provide some measure of the timing of an ischaemic event.

The volume of early necrosis marks only the central volume of a stroke. The surrounding area of reduced flow (which can be substantial) remains at risk of later irreversible damage. The extent of ultimate tissue damage is a function both of the degree of flow reduction and the time for which this flow reduction is maintained. The area of reduced flow around the necrotic core therefore defines the potentially salvageable 'ischaemic penumbra'. This tissue is a major target of therapeutic interventions. The combined use of diffusion and perfusion MR imaging can be used to define the ischaemic penumbra. Perfusion images have been generated most commonly using a gadolinium-bolus tracking method in which the signal change on a T1-weighted image after injection of gadolinium-DTPA is followed with time. More recently the methodology has been extended with use of entirely non-invasive 'arterial spin-tagging'.[2] While both of these methods are most commonly used in a qualitative way, providing an index of relative decreases in flow, advances in methodology promise that quantitation may be possible.

These approaches are complemented by MR angiographic techniques which can localize areas of arterial occlusion. Advances in imaging technology, particularly with higher-field magnets, may allow medium and small vessels to be imaged with this technique. There remain problems with interpretation of areas of signal loss associated with turbulence in the MR angiographic image, but these are more critical for defining quantitative indices of the extent of occlusion than they are in identifying points of occlusion.

More conventional imaging technology based on T2-weighted imaging has also advanced. These techniques are in general most useful for assessment of load of disease. Approaches such as FLAIR imaging have proved much more sensitive to ischaemic white matter changes than standard T2-imaging. With the use of fast spin-echo imaging sequences, the time for acquisition of data has also decreased, allowing a much thinner slice of data to be acquired and thereby also potentially increasing the sensitivity with which lesion volumes can be defined, particularly for diffuse (i.e. multi-focal) disease.

An exciting new development in MRI has been functional magnetic resonance imaging.[3] This technique utilizes signal changes dependent on local alterations of blood flow and blood oxygenation accompanying neuronal activation of areas of brain involved in specific cognitive processes such as movement, language production, or sensation. These techniques have been used in the normal brain to finely map the cortical (and, more recently, sub-cortical) areas involved in these tasks. As the methods do not involve injection of radioactive materials they can be used easily in serial follow-up of patients.

In initial applications of FMRI to stroke, it has become clear that patients with infarcts affecting motor pathways generate movement with use of multiple parallel pathways that normally are not used in this way. Recruitment of ipsilateral motor cortex, increased recruitment of contralateral motor cortex around the area of damage, and also changes in contralateral pre-motor and supplementary motor cortex activation have been seen. Applications have also been demonstrated in studies of patients with aphasia and in those with 'blindsight', in which directed but unconscious responses to visual stimuli can be demonstrated after injury to the primary visual cortex.

Magnetic resonance spectroscopy can be used to provide information on the biochemistry of tissue damage.[4] Early changes in lactic levels are a sensitive index of an anaerobic metabolism. Injury to axons and axonal loss or neuronal loss can be assessed by decreases in the neuronal-specific marker, N-acetylaspartate. A good relationship has been shown between the extent of disability and the extent of decreases in this molecule in patients post-stroke. Finally, inflammatory or membrane changes may be localized using changes in the molecule choline.

Parallel with developments in data acquisition have been improvements in image analysis. One application has been for defining the axonal injury that appears to be an important proximate of mechanism for disability in a broad range of central nervous system insults. Axonal injury is associated with loss of volume, particularly of periventricular white matter. Sensitive image analysis methods based on the registration of serial images allow small changes (even of the order of 1%) to be defined in brain volume. These techniques have already been demonstrated as surrogate markers of progressive disease in neurodegenerative disorders such as Alzheimer's disease, suggesting that their application to chronically progressive, multifocal stroke may also be useful.

Serial registration and subtraction of images can be used to define, very sensitively, changes in lesion size. The registration of images from the same individuals at different times can be done with sub-pixel accuracy. Subtraction images generated from this registration provide sensitive markers of changes in lesion loads.[5] These can be quantified by objective, threshold-based methods, allowing precise measurement of changes in lesion load. Serial monitoring in multiple sclerosis is sensitive to changes arising from therapeutic interventions. The potential of the networks for long-term monitoring of patients with micro-vascular stroke or for monitoring of changes in individual stroke lesions over time is also high.

The spatial distribution of lesions and differences in lesion distribution with specific groups can be defined by MR using image analysis techniques based on group analysis. The development of probabilistic lesion distribution maps (or 'lesion probability maps') has been used in multiple sclerosis to define the nature of micro-vascular lesions across populations. This may be useful in helping to subcategorize stroke syndromes.

A major challenge in both treatment and in the evaluation of new treatments is to adequately define populations with homogenous pathologies. It is likely that defining such sub-populations may be critical for appropriate targeting of therapies. As expensive new treatments become available, it is imperative to target them to the population that will draw the most benefit. MR techniques that can provide more detailed information on the nature of the underlying pathology should provide important tools for doing this, particularly as the techniques become efficient and more appropriate for use immediately on presentation.

References

1. Albers, G. W. (1998). Diffusion-weighted MRI for evaluation of acute stroke. *Neurology*, **51**, S47–9.
2. Jezzard, P. (1998). Advances in perfusion imaging. *Radiology*, **208**, 296–9.
3. Matthews, P. M., Clare, S., Adcock, J. Functional magnetic resonance imaging: clinical applications and potential. *J. Inherit. Metab. Dis.* **22**, 337–52.
4. Arnold, D., Matthews, P. M. (1995). Focal brain lesions in human MRS. In: *Encylopedia of nuclear magnetic resonance* (ed. D. M. Grant, R. K. Harris). Wiley, London.
5. Lee, M. A., Smith, S., Palace, J., Matthews, P. M. (1998). Defining multiple sclerosis disease activity using T2-weighted difference imaging. *Brain*, **121**, 2095–102.

Section 6

Therapy and rehabilitation

18   Evolution and revolution in speech and language therapy

PROFESSOR PAM ENDERBY

Chair of Community Rehabilitation
Centre for Ageing and Rehabilitation Studies, University of Sheffield

Context

Approximately one-third of the patients who survive a stroke will have an obvious speech or language difficulty. It is suspected that many more have more subtle difficulties associated with comprehension and/or expression, which may have an impact on their future lives. Whilst the most common disorder associated with a single stroke is that of dysphasia, where the person may have difficulty in understanding written or spoken speech or expressing themselves fully and coherently, there are many who have a motor speech disorder which is commonly associated with either bilateral or brain-stem strokes. Motor speech disorders may be related to dysarthria or dyspraxia and result in the individual having difficulty in articulating words clearly.[1] Persons with dysphasia, dysarthria, or dyspraxia may have mild difficulties, making communication slightly frustrating and irritating, or may be left without the ability to communicate even basic needs and wants.

In addition to speech and language disorders, many patients following stroke may also have a swallowing disorder – dysphagia – which

---

Dysphasia   A language disorder which can cause difficulties both in expressing and comprehending speech, written language, and gesture.

Dysarthria   A motor speech difficulty leading to the inability to articulate any sounds or a disturbance in articulation resulting in slurred, distorted, and abnormal sounding speech.

Dyspraxia   A motor programming disorder leading to difficulty in planning and controlling motor speech and resulting in difficulty in imitating and producing speech in a consistent manner.

more recently has attracted the attention of speech and language therapists who are now integrally involved in its assessment and management.

Speech and language therapists have worked with persons with dysphasia and dysarthria since the First World War, and in fact it was these disorders that were catalytic in developing their profession. However, there appear to have been different themes and approaches to the rehabilitation of those with communication deficits and these are addressed below.

Development of speech and language therapy

An early theme of the approach to speech and language therapy was to assess the specific aspects of the language disorder and to treat those aspects of difficulty by structuring tasks in a progressive way, aiming to assist people to relearn these skills. A later approach was where the retained abilities of the patient were seen as the focus of therapy, and speech and language therapists developed programmes that exploited retained communication skills. Surprisingly, it was not until the 1970s that a greater emphasis was placed on the importance of developing functional communication, that is, not teaching patients to use words or sounds but assisting them with communicating more effectively in general, be it through gesture, drawing, or any other means.

At this time the debate in speech and language therapy was related to whether general stimulation improves the communication of dysphasic patients, i.e. if one can motivate a patient to try and communicate and give them every opportunity to speak, does this practice lead to overall improvements? This was found to be the case in most research studies. General language stimulation, whether given by a speech and language therapist or an untrained volunteer, was found to be effective as compared to people who did not have such encouragement or attention. In the 1980s the speech and language therapists became more aware that teaching patients strategies to overcome their problems might be more effective, and thus in the last 15 years there have been many studies exploring the underlying psycholinguistic, i.e. the psychological aspects of communication, and the neurolinguistic, i.e. the neurophysiological and neurological, components of language. This led to speculation about the different aspects of the language process and whether disruption at different points in this process results in predictable symptoms. There is now a better understanding of the different skills underpinning language, which has led to exploration of hypotheses being captured within therapy. Thus, the treatment of choice currently is more specific, targeted treatments based on the individual patient's linguistic deficits. Research in this area has established that this strategic approach to language therapy appears to be more effective than general stimulation alone.[2]

However, we now come to a strange division of emphasis by speech and language therapists. In the mid to late 1980s some speech and language therapists felt that this approach to remediation was entirely appropriate for individuals with speech and language disorders, whereas others felt that it was inappropriate to remediate the disorder itself without thinking of the person in broader ways and ensuring that a more holistic approach was taken to the rehabilitation programme. In the 1990s a healthy combination has been embedded into the present practice of speech and language therapy with a greater acknowledgement that the impairment needs a specialist-specific and fairly intensive approach which is likely to be a 'functionally relevant process', whilst at the same time ensuring that patients and their relatives are assisted to communicate in the most effective way. Furthermore, there is an improved understanding about the impact of speech and language disorders on social participation and the general well-being of individual clients and their families. Unfortunately, at the time when we have greatest knowledge about the procedures that can specifically help people regain language skills and a better understanding of how we can improve interactive and effective communication, there appears to be a reduction in the resources available to provide speech and language therapy. We now have evidence that the impact of dysphagia on the workloads of speech and language therapists has directly reduced the amount of time they have available to treat those with dysphasia,[3] despite the fact that there possibly is less evidence for the unique contribution that they can make with dysphagia and improving confidence with regard to the profession and its treatment of dysphagia. So we enter the new millennium with a new issue to debate and a new set of challenges. It is important that those patients with dysphagia get appropriate care; whether this is by speech and language therapists on their own or working with others needs to be addressed urgently. We also need to ensure that organizers and purchasers of services are confident that the profession has progressed a long way with regard to the evidence relating to the role of communication therapy within rehabilitation, and we must defend this role and resource.

The future

So what are the challenges to speech and language therapy in the next two decades? Firstly we have to address the issue of resources. The majority of patients who acquire a speech and language disorder receive less than 45 minutes per week of therapy treatment for a post-stroke three-month period. Wondering whether something so thinly spread is effective or not seems rather an arid debate. We have to consider whether the skills of the speech and language therapists should be diverted to the management of dysphagia or whether there are other ways of handling that disorder but preserving the appropriate use of skills of the profession. One possible solution is to use computers to assist with the administration and support of speech and language therapy. In the Speech and Language Therapy Research Unit we have been conducting research on supplemented therapy over a ten-year period. This has allowed us a glimpse into the future. We have already established that older patients who have had no previous experience of computers are able to use them readily and like doing so. We have also found that some of the tasks undertaken on the computer will generalize to other functional settings, and while we need to conduct further research in this area, early indications are promising. Many of the people who are involved in our research use their computers for many hours a week, something that is not found to be the case when doing traditional speech and language therapy 'homework'. We have also established that many post-stroke patients can be involved in specific treatment exercises which they find rewarding and stimulating.

An area that excites me for the future is monitoring progress in a more appropriate fashion. Many of the dysphasia tests are long, convoluted, and require sophisticated analysis. Unfortunately, because of their complexity, they are used infrequently and often not in the most scientifically sound manner. However, a computer can sample a patient's performance readily on frequent occasions, allowing good insight instead of just assessment in a snap-shot fashion.

There are several areas of challenge for the future: to establish the appropriate use of speech and language therapy resources by improving our accuracy in identifying which patients will benefit from which treatments; to supplement treatment by exploiting the use of computer technology for the benefit of patients; to continue to investigate the psycholinguistic and neurolinguistic principles of speech that underpin much of the promising areas of the treatment of impairment; and to explore how we can best equip those with dysphasia to live life to the full whilst being challenged with one of the most socially compromising of deficits.[4]

There is evidence that attending to dysphagia reduces mortality and morbidity. There is also equal evidence that attending to the communication disorders of patients can, with some, improve the specific impairment, and in others affect functional communication and improve social participation and the quality of life. The challenges in the future will be to ensure that we can close the gap between what research indicates and what services can provide.

References

1. Chapman, S. B. (1991). Aphasia and ageing. In: *Geriatric communication disorders* (ed. D. Rippich), pp. 241–55. Proed, Texas.
2. Enderby, P., Emerson, J. (1995). *Does speech and language therapy work: A review of the literature*, pp. 11–34. Singular Publishing, London.
3. Enderby, P., Petheram, B. (1998). Changes in referral to speech and language therapy. *Int. J. Lang. Comm. Dis.*, 33(Suppl.), 16–21.
4. Byng, S., Black, M. (1995). What makes a therapy? Some parameters of therapeutic intervention. *Eur. J. Dis. Comm.*, 30, 303–16.

19   Motor control following stroke

DR ANN ASHBURN

MSc Course Coordinator/Senior Lecturer in Rehabilitation
Southampton General Hospital

Introduction

Movement disorders following stroke are common and the treatment of patients with motor problems forms a major work commitment for many physiotherapists in hospitals and community rehabilitation settings. The re-education of motor control and functional ability are the main targets for treatment by therapists who may use a combination of observational, verbal, manual, and educational skills. Deficits of movement, abnormalities of tone, and sensation can influence the initiation and quality of voluntary movement and postural control. Although physiotherapy is likely to be only one of several components in a rehabilitation programme, physical recovery will probably dominate the expectations of patients, staff, and family at the expense of cognitive, emotional, and social factors.[1] Rising costs of stroke management, variability of the consequences of stroke, and need for effective services have driven the search for effective management programmes, ways of identifying rehabilitation potential, and greater understanding of movement recovery. Nearly all individuals with stroke receive some type of rehabilitation so predicting the outcome is complex – it encompasses the combined effect of natural recovery, responsiveness of individuals to therapy, and effectiveness of the treatment procedure.

Recovery of movement

Evidence indicates that recovery is most rapid in the first few months with patterns of movement recurring in similar hierarchy in most patients, although there are exceptions. The initial level of motor dysfunction and the time interval between paralysis and return of movement have been reported as important indicators of the recovery process. The prognostic importance of balance control in sitting in the acute stage has been recognized by several researchers. Morgan[2] found that static sitting balance within 48 hours of an acute stroke correlated positively with an independent gait at six weeks. Laterality of lesion has not been shown to significantly influence the final outcome, but studies of cognition have identified links between unilateral neglect and poor function. Interestingly there is a paucity of work on the long-term sequelae of movement disorders following stroke. In particular, changes in movement dysfunction over time in severely dependent subjects and in those who make a rapid recovery have not been reported.

Treatment approaches

In the past decade there have been significant advances in the development of models of motor control from a physiotherapeutic perspective.[3] These models have helped develop a framework for the current physiotherapeutic approaches used in the retraining of movement. The approaches have evolved from the work of pioneers such as Bobath, Kabat, Peto, and Carr and Shepherd.[3] Although these approaches are widely thought to be contradictory, there are many common features, not least the aim to improve motor control. Key differences between the approaches centre around the amount, type, and basis for applying sensory stimuli in the facilitation of motor learning. Most clinicians do not follow a single approach in a purist manner, even though they are likely to favour one.

To date, research into the treatment of movement problems has been directed primarily at identifying which of the physiotherapy approaches is optimal, but multiple clinical studies have demonstrated no clear difference between them in effectiveness. Evidence shows that patients derive benefit from the provision of organized rehabilitation, including physiotherapy, and that treatment with any of the available approaches will improve the patient's functional status. Deficiencies in research designs though have compromised the quality of many studies and could explain the equivocal findings.[4]

Other researchers have examined particular features of interventions such as the effects of training-specific tasks, varying intensity of physiotherapy, and muscle-strength training. Findings illustrate limited transfer of task skills to other activities, a small but positive effect of increase in intensity, and beneficial effects of muscle-strength training in selected subjects.

Interactive process

Movement retraining is concerned with more than the manual techniques used and the educational principles followed by physiotherapists. The attributes of patients are key to the process of intervention which is interactive and directed by the responses of individuals. There is little written about what guides judgements and clinical decisions made by therapists, but there is a growing body of knowledge about the influence of empowerment and inner belief on outcome and recovery.[5] Also, increasing numbers of researchers are examining the content of therapy programmes in order to try to understand the process of intervention.

Conclusion

In conclusion, stroke patients benefit from organized rehabilitation, including physiotherapy, but the optimal approach has yet to be identified. Future studies need to seek information from patients and therapists in order to develop a comprehensive understanding of the range of patient responses to therapy techniques and training programmes. The theoretical framework for practice must continue to develop in order to allow therapists to make clinical decisions based on evidence and not myths.

References

1. Forster, A., Young, J. (1992). Stroke rehabilitation. Can we do better? *Br. Med. J.*, **305**, 1446–7.
2. Morgan, P. (1994). The relationship between sitting balance and mobility outcome in stroke. *Aus. Physio.*, **40**(2), 91–6.
3. Plant, R. (1998). Treatment approaches in neurological rehabilitation. In: *Neurological physiotherapy* (ed. M. Stokes). Mosby, London.
4. Ashburn, A., Powtridge, C., DeSouza, L. (1993). Physiotherapy in the rehabilitation of stroke: A review. *Clin. Rehab.*, **7**, 337–45.
5. Zimmerman, M., Warschautsky, S. (1998). Empowerment theory for rehabilitation research: Conceptual and methodological issues. *Rehab. Psychol.*, **43**(I), 3–16.

20 Occupational therapy

DR AVRIL DRUMMOND

Senior Occupational Therapist/Research Officer
University of Nottingham

The last 100 years has been a time of great development for occupational therapy (OT) as well as for The Stroke Association. The term 'occupational therapy' has only been used since the beginning of this century and, since then, there has been recognition as a profession, the formation of an association, and state registration.

Today OT is recognized as an important part of rehabilitation, particularly with those who have had a stroke. However, it is only in the last decade or so that emphasis has been placed on the need for research. Benefits of stroke rehabilitation packages (including OT) have already been demonstrated in several studies. However, it is not known what the individual contribution of OT was in these packages. It is only in recent years that researchers have examined specific OT treatments.

Two trials have examined specific techniques used in OT. Drummond and Walker randomly allocated 65 patients who had had a stroke into three groups (two treatment, one control).[1] They found that the group who had received leisure treatment intervention had better leisure scores than the other groups. In another study, 30 patients with dressing problems post stroke had a sustained reduction in this after receiving dressing practice.[2]

Other studies have compared a global OT package with a control situation. Logan *et al.* randomly allocated 111 patients to receive either conventional social services input or enhanced input.[3] At three months' follow-up the group receiving extra treatment had better extended activities of daily living scores. Another study offered an additional six weeks of OT to patients in their treatment group.[4] The researchers found that at seven weeks' follow-up the treatment group had improved functional scores. Results of the six months' follow-up are awaited.

Although all of these and other studies had positive results, relatively small numbers of patients were included in the trials and much longer-term evaluation is needed to see if benefits were maintained. Also, all of the patients in these studies were recruited after discharge from hospital. Walker *et al.* have just reported a study of 185 non-hospitalized stroke patients who were randomly allocated to receive OT or not.[5] At six months' follow-up there were significant differences between the groups on functional scores and differences on the Carer Strain Index in favour of the treatment group.

Unfortunately, although the results from these trials are promising, they still leave many fundamental questions unanswered. For example, most basic of all is the question 'What is occupational therapy?'. Very little has actually been documented about what occupational therapists do in treatment sessions with their patients. In addition to studying the content of OT, we need long-term evaluation of specific approaches. It is interesting to note how many routine treatments are used which have never been examined. For example, there has been a long-running debate within the profession about the preferred method of treating perceptual problems. Some therapists have advocated a functional approach, while others support the use of the transfer of training approach. A recent Nottingham study comparing the two approaches showed no differences at six weeks.

Work is needed in many other areas. Among the priorities must be targeting those stroke patients who respond best to treatment, evaluating the best places for treatment, and examining cost implications. We also need to study the timing as well as the delivery of treatment. Most importantly, research must become an integral part of day-to-day practice. Occupational therapists who do research often have to leave a clinical post to pursue a research interest, and this can set up barriers within the profession. Doctors are actively encouraged to do research, and therapists must be given the same encouragement, support, and opportunities.

References

1. Drummond, A. E., Walker, M. F. (1995). A randomized controlled trial of leisure rehabilitation after stroke. *Clin. Rehab.*, 9, 283–90.
2. Walker, M. F., Drummond, A. E., Lincoln, N. B. (1996). Evaluation of dressing practice for stroke patients after discharge from hospital: a cross-over design study. *Clin. Rehab.*, 10, 23–31.
3. Logan, P. A., Ahern, J., Gladman, J. R. F., Lincoln, N. B. (1997). A randomized controlled trial of enhanced social service occupational therapy for stroke patients. *Clin. Rehab.*, 11, 107–13.

4. Gilbertson, L., Langhorne, P., Walker, A., Allen, A. (1998). A randomized controlled trial of home-based occupational therapy for stroke patients: results at 7 weeks [abstract]. *Cerebrovasc. Dis.*, 8(4), 84.
5. Walker, M. F., Gladman, J. R. F., Lincoln, N. B., Siemonsma, P., Whiteley, T. A randomized controlled trial of occupational therapy for stroke patients not admitted to hospital. (Submitted for publication.)

21   Future approaches to stroke rehabilitation

PROFESSOR RAY TALLIS

Professor of Geriatric Medicine
Hope Hospital, Salford

There is an increasing body of evidence that rehabilitation is effective following stroke. It is one of the key elements of stroke units, which are known not only to save lives but also to reduce disability[1] – an effect that is sustained in the long term.[2] There is some evidence that this beneficial effect is at least in part due to rehabilitation, in as much as there appears to be a dose-dependent effect – more rehabilitation is associated with a better functional outcome.[3]

There are, however, no grounds for complacency. Many stroke patients still remain seriously disabled, and indeed dependent, and may be institutionalized after a stroke. Even those who make a 'good' recovery often experience difficulties in psychosocial reintegration. The art of stroke rehabilitation is relatively undeveloped as a science.

For a start, we do not have a clear idea of the components of the 'package' that are bringing about the modest benefits that are seen. We have little knowledge of how much of the benefit is due to the specific rehabilitation techniques of physical remediation and how much is due to more general measures such as counselling, education, advice, and the provision of aids and adaptations. We are even further from having a clear idea as to which of the various techniques of physical remediation are most effective, and from identifying the components of those approaches that might be most powerful in driving recovery. Indeed, we have little information about the actual procedures included in various therapy techniques. Moreover, there has been little or no detailed evaluation of the contributions made by the different disciplines to the outcome of stroke care. In summary, stroke therapy is a long way from being rooted in neuroscience.

There are several ways forward. Better and more imaginative use of devices for helping patients to interact with the physical environment – orthoses, prostheses, and environmental control systems – and new approaches to psychological reintegration, based upon a deeper understanding of why some patients with relatively mild impairments do badly and others with severe impairments do well, are two strategies that should be explored in depth. Nevertheless, although they could well produce worthwhile gains, it seems unlikely that these strategies will bring dramatic improvements in our ability to restore patients to independence and freedom. A more attractive strategy is to look at ways in which impairments themselves might be reversed.

There are two major strands to this strategy. The first will be to evaluate current techniques of therapy with a view to identifying those elements that seem to be most effective, evaluating them using appropriate measures, and trying to build on their effects by, for example, increasing the 'dose' of treatment. In view of the complexity of therapies, this is likely to be rather laborious and may yield limited returns.[4] The second, more promising strand, will be to develop novel therapies based on a more deliberate and effective exploitation of what is known about the mechanisms of recovery and about those factors that drive recovery, with the intention of promoting adaptive plastic changes and inhibiting maladaptive ones.

There is an increasing body of research testifying to the extraordinary capacity of the nervous system to reorganize in changing input response to direct damage[5] or in response to changing input due to more peripheral damage.[6] This has supported the notion that the structure and function of the nervous system is maintained and shaped by information derived from the experience associated with normal activity. Recent imaging techniques have shown this in considerable detail.[7] A biological plausible research strategy will therefore be to try to drive recovery by inputing the equivalent of this activity-derived information either by (a) using assisted activity, or (b) alternative methods such as carefully designed electrotherapies[8-10] or other modalities of stimulation to deliver 'prosthetic experience'. Assisted activity as deployed in the future may not seem radically different from the conventional therapy currently available. However, it will differ in at least two respects: the dose will be adequate rather than homoeopathic and the treatment will be customized to deficits that are more precisely characterized in neurophysiological or neuropsychological terms. Electrotherapies and other ways of delivering 'prosthetic experience' will exploit not only emerging neuroscientific understanding but also new electronic and computational technologies to a degree not hitherto seen in rehabilitation.

These new approaches will take a long time to develop. It will be a sign of the scientific maturity of neurotherapy that practitioners will no longer expect the overnight emergence of new techniques, and instant solutions as to how to treat patients (attached to the name of a charismatic leader of a particular school) will be treated with suspicion. Improvement in the effectiveness of neurotherapy will be incremental. Relatively slow progress will be likely not only because of the technological challenge, but also because genuinely scientifically-based treatments will be predicated upon a more thorough teasing out and delineation of deficits, so that treatments will – at least initially – be evaluated on relatively homogeneous groups of patients or patients with 'pure' or 'focal' lesions. Moreover, evaluation of the effectiveness of new treatments will require outcome measures that will be addressed to more clearly defined hypotheses as to the putative neurophysiological effects of treatment. This will demand the invention of new measurement tools and these, more often than not, will be physical instruments rather than the often unilluminating scales and indices that have figured so largely in the rehabilitation literature of the last few decades.

Developing better therapies for stroke patients will require a huge effort. This has major implications for the way stroke rehabilitation research should be planned and organized. The contrast between the 'cottage industries' supporting research into therapies and the massive infrastructure underpinning the development and production of science-based pharmaceutical treatments is striking. This will need to be redressed if rehabilitation research is going to proceed at the rate our patients are entitled to expect.

The future of stroke rehabilitation is potentially very exciting but the commitment to rooting neurotherapy in neuroscience may require a major change in mind-set. However, it is important that the gains of the last few decades in the care and support of stroke patients are not lost. Science-based therapeutic techniques will always remain only a part of the art, craft, and humanity of care that is necessary if we are to limit the damage inflicted on peoples' lives by stroke.

References

1. Stroke Unit Trialists' Collaboration (1997). Collaborative systematic review of organised in-patient (stroke unit) care after stroke. *Br. Med. J.*, **314**, 1151–9.
2. Indredarvik, B., Bakke, F., Slordahl, S. A., Rokseth, R., Haheim, L. L. (1997). Stroke unit treatment: Long-term effects. *Stroke*, **28**, 1861–6.
3. Kwakkel, G., Wagenaar, R. C., Koelman, T. W., Lankhorst, G. J., Koestsier, J. C. (1997). Effect of intensity of rehabilitation after stroke. *Stroke*, **28**, 1550–6.

4. Pomeroy, V. M., Niven, D. S., Faragher, E. B., Tallis, R. C. (1999). Unpacking the black box of nursing and therapy practice for post-stroke shoulder pain: a necessary precursor to evaluation. *Cerebrovasc. Dis.*, **9**, 28.

5. Hallet, M., Wasserman, E., Coehn, L. G., Chmielowska, J., Gerloff, C. (1998). Cortical mechanisms of recovery of function after stroke. *Neurorehabilitation*, **10**, 131–42.

6. Hamdy, S., Aziz, Q., Rothwell, J. C., Singh, K., Barlow, J., Hughes, D. G., *et al.* (1996). The cortical topography of swallowing motor function in man. *Nat. Med.*, **2**(11), 1217–24.

7. Frackowiak, R. S. J. (1996). Plasticity and the human brain: insights from functional imaging. *Neuroscientist*, **2**, 353–62.

8. Prada, G. O., Tallis, R. C. (1995). Treatment of the neglect syndrome in stroke patients using a contingency electrical stimulator. *Clin. Rehab.*, **9**, 77–86.

9. Smith, L. E. (1990). Restoration of volitional limb movement of hemiplegics following patterned functional electrical stimulation. *Percept. Mot. Skills*, **71**, 851–61.

10. Hamdy, S., Rothwell, J. C., Aziz, Q., Singh, K. D., Thompson, D. G. (1998). Long-term reorganization of human motor cortex driven by short-term sensory stimulation. *Nat. Neurosci.*, **1**, 64–8.

Section 7
Stroke and stroke care

22   Stroke care: a matter of chance

PROFESSOR SHAH EBRAHIM AND
JUDITH REDFERN

MRC Health Services Research Collaboration
University of Bristol and Royal Free and
University College Medical School, London

Background

Stroke is the third most common cause of death in the UK and is the most common cause of severe disability. Organized stroke services have been widely evaluated and are an effective means of reducing death, disability, and institutional placement following acute stroke.[1] There is a growing awareness of the need to improve the quality of stroke services and to implement organized stroke services more widely. A Stroke Association survey conducted in 1992/93 found that such services were not widespread.[2]

Objective

Our objective was to obtain national data on stroke services (structure, operational policies and practices, research and audit, and planning) to act as a benchmark against which current standards can be audited.

Design

Two national surveys were undertaken, one of all consultants in the UK responsible for the care of stroke patients to provide hospital data on services, and one of all health authorities and health boards in the UK to provide data on commissioning of stroke services.

Response rates

A total of 2954 (80%) consultants returned questionnaires, and 73% completed a questionnaire. Of these, 1716 (58%) cared for stroke patients. A total of 103 (82%) out of 124 health authorities and health boards completed questionnaires.

Definition

Organized stroke services are provided by interdisciplinary teams in hospitals, usually working in a geographically defined stroke unit. Occasionally such teams care for stroke patients throughout a hospital without a defined stroke unit. Features distinguishing such services from general medical services are coordinated interdisciplinary care, involvement of family and carers in the rehabilitation process, specialization, and education of staff, patients, and carers.[1]

Main findings

The majority of stroke patients are managed by consultants in general medical specialties (54%) and geriatric medicine (27%). Only 44 (3%) consultants looking after stroke patients identified themselves as specialists in stroke medicine. The number of patients managed by consultants from different specialties varies widely, with geriatricians and stroke medicine specialists responsible, on average, for nine and 15 patients respectively on the day of the survey.

Over three-quarters of consultants have access to organized stroke services, although approximately half of stroke patients do not get into them. This results in between 4500 and 7000 avoidable deaths and institutional placements every year, of which deaths account for just under half.

Despite an overall improvement in access since 1992/93, there is wide and unacceptable variation around the UK in the chances of being managed in an organized stroke service. Patients in Northern Ireland, Scotland, and Wales are approximately twice as likely to be managed by organized stroke services as patients in England. Patients in the south-west region of England are only half as likely to be managed by organized stroke services as patients in the rest of the UK.

The patients of only a third of consultants are usually managed in a stroke unit or by a stroke team, resulting in only half of stroke patients receiving optimal specialist stroke services. Social work support is a particular concern with over a third (36.7%) of consultants stating that social workers provided inadequate time for their patients. Many consultants experience delays in the organization of community services – social services home care (meals, home help) took over a week to arrange according to half the consultants surveyed. Few services can be arranged speedily, resulting in patients waiting in hospital unnecessarily.

Access to neuroradiology remains difficult. Provision of CT scanning has improved but urgent access still appears to be difficult. Only just over a third (37%) of consultants said they were able to get a CT scan for their patients the same or next day after admission. Urgent CT scanning will be essential should a safe and effective acute stroke treatment be found. Hospitals will have to work out how to provide a 24-hour neuroradiology service for stroke patients.

Consultants are fairly well informed about the benefits and hazards of specific acute and preventive treatments for stroke. Most (74–85%) were uncertain of the effects of low-molecular-weight heparin and thrombolytic therapies. Ninety per cent of stroke patients are admitted within 24 hours of onset, which allows accurate diagnosis and supportive treatments to be used early.

Consultants considered stroke rehabilitation units to be very valuable (66%), and also considered other services very valuable – acute stroke units (18.4%), family support workers (23.7%), community stroke teams (27.6%), transient ischaemic attack (TIA)/rapid OPD (out patient department) (39.3%). There was more uncertainty about these latter services, reflecting the limited evidence for them. Commissioners of health services are also sure of the value of stroke units, both acute and rehabilitation, but were less convinced of the value of combined acute/rehabilitation units, family support workers, and TIA/rapid OPD.

Levels of audit and research in stroke are surprisingly high with over half of consultants reporting an audit and a third carrying out research in the last five years. These activities have direct benefits to patients who will be more likely to receive standardized care, regular assessment, and follow-up.

Only 3% of those looking after stroke patients are specialists in stroke medicine. These consultants were more likely to be well informed about local policies, use standard assessment protocols, provide patient information, perform research and audit, and organize in-service staff training than other consultants. Promotion of specialists in stroke medicine is not a priority for health service commissioners.

Consultants are working in an information and policy vacuum. Just under half (42%) of consultants reported that a written stroke strategy existed, while only a fifth had defined minimum standards of care. Opportunities to improve services through written strategies, contracting, minimum care standards, and training are being missed. These gaps are a reflection of a lack of leadership in stroke services.

Stroke is certainly viewed as a priority for district service commissioners. However, there is a variable approach to commissioning with both specific stroke services or general acute and rehabilitation services being used. The current organization of services means that stroke services are commissioned in a piecemeal fashion which makes integration difficult.

Conclusions

Variation in access to, and use of, stroke services is unacceptable and requires urgent action by health service commissioners. Better information and management tools are required for both consultants and health service commissioners. The lack of basic information on numbers of stroke patients and costs of care makes planning services difficult. Stronger medical leadership is required. The development of a new sub-specialty of stroke medicine might improve leadership, organization, and service planning, leading to better patient care.

References

1. Stroke Unit Trialists' Collaboration (1997). Collaborative systematic review of the randomised trials of organised in-patient (stroke unit) care after stroke. *Br. Med. J.*, **314**, 1151–9.
2. Lindley, R., Amayo, E., Marshall, J., Sandercock, P., Dennis, M., Warlow, C. P. (1995). Hospital services for patients with acute stroke in the UK: The Stroke Association survey of consultant opinion. *Age Ageing*, **24**, 525–32.

23

The quality of stroke service provision

PROFESSOR M. SEVERS

Professor in Elderly Health Care
Queen Alexandra Hospital, Portsmouth

Service provision is a system of supplying a public need.[1] There is no standard in the NHS for assessing whole systems, nor indeed for building them, as in service development. Quality is multidimensional and is usually defined as the degree to which health services for individuals and populations increase the likelihood of desired health outcomes and are consistent with current professional knowledge.[2] In assessing the quality of a stroke service one is therefore required to examine not only the patients who receive certain interventions, but also those who do not but who are nevertheless in need. The Clinical Standards Advisory Group (CSAG) set up a study in 1996 into clinical effectiveness using stroke care as an example, which enabled the research team to not only investigate individual interventions, but also how they fitted together into a service. This paper highlights a number of areas, some of which were published in the CSAG report of 1998.[3] Caring for people with stroke illness is a human activity system, i.e. human beings undertaking purposeful activity.[4] The assessment of the quality of service provision has therefore been approached from a systems thinking and systems practice perspective.[5,6]

The first step in assessing a stroke service is to be clear about the customer or who the service is for. The target population needs to be identified so that each component of the service can be designed to meet their needs. This is important for patients who may not get access to effective services like stroke units[7] because the rehabilitation unit was not designed to meet patient need but was simply built to the size that seemed reasonable to the local space, resource, and preference. Only one out of the nine stroke units found in the sample of seven districts visited had any evidence that the stroke unit had been designed to meet the numbers in need of such a service. This is also important for the practitioners themselves as they are increasingly being assessed externally by a variety of performance management techniques.[8] Lack of clarity about the patients in the service

may give spurious results about the quality of service due to variations in the severity of stroke and the presence of complicating and
non-complicating comorbidities.[9] The ability to use routine data
for quality assessment is limited by terming (record keeping) and
classifying (coding) imperfections as well as by case-mix adjustment
problems.

Lastly, lack of clarity about patient characteristics can impair the
movements of patients between service components. A failure to
have a clear understanding of which stroke patients should be admitted means some patients are not being admitted when they should be
and vice versa. It also means multiple assessment and indecision
when none is necessary. In one district two guidelines were found
which differed in their recommendations on who to admit; others
failed to be clinically specific.

The environments of care are of critical importance in the care of
stroke patients, but they are rarely synthesized into a patient experience within a service. When this is done it begins to create a picture
of environmental changes which calls into question some service
configurations. There are four possible environments which stroke
patients referred by GP encounter when they reach hospital:

(1) accident and emergency   3/15 (20%);
(2) medical assessment unit   7/15 (47%);
(3) acute stroke unit   2/15 (13%);
(4) general wards   3/15 (20%).

However, this static picture does not give insight into patient
movements with time. In the first week a hospitalized stroke victim
can expect three moves in 60% of hospitals when the admission is
via accident and emergency, and in 53% of hospitals when the admission is via the GP. Two trusts offered direct access to GPs to their
acute stroke unit and reported no problems at all. Equally, stroke
rehabilitation units were found in teaching hospitals, district general
hospitals, community hospitals, and geriatric medicine hospitals –
although they appear equally effective clinically, the costs of each
environment is very different and each has different access characteristics for the patients' relatives. As patient preferences become more
prominent in health service delivery, environmental factors are likely
to become much higher on the agenda of service planning.

Audit is the most common evaluation method of stroke services; it
tends to focus on the transformation process. This is the term that
encompasses the activities or interventions of the service. From five

districts only 14 audits could be found relating to stroke. These 14 were nearly all in secondary care and only eight of them included any results; there were no re-audits. Other contributors have dealt with most of the important evidence-based interventions, but it is important to recognize that there is a lack of evidence in many areas crucial for clinical effectiveness. These gaps are either complete gaps, for example in many areas around the management of dysphagia, or partial gaps. Partial gaps are the knowledge deficits between efficacy (those interventions proven in research) and effectiveness (those interventions proven in practice). They are very important at the service assessment level. For example, anticoagulation has benefits in both primary and secondary prevention in patients with chronic non-rheumatic atrial fibrillation.[10,11] The extent to which it is effective in practice depends on the local bleed rate – none of the medical staff interviewed in the CSAG study and only 17% of respondents to questionnaires knew the local haemorrhagic complication rates. Given published haemorrhage rates in practice of between 2.8% and 11%,[12–15] the margin of benefit and harm in any given setting is uncomfortably thin, especially for primary prevention. The key is knowledge of the local haemorrhage rate, which is not present in many services.

The staffing of a service is crucial to its quality. Despite this statement of the obvious there is no standard or template for staffing in terms of stroke care. Given that about 70% of the costs of running a service is staffing, it is surprising that more progress has not been made. The CSAG study did look at staffing, particularly in units which were called 'stroke units' by the staff in the visit sites. Staffing variations were very large, as shown in Table 23.1.

There is much work to do in increasing both our understanding and practice around staffing and its relationships with the quality of stroke services. At present staffing is not driven by evidence, national consensus, nor by the case-mix of the patients.

For a stroke service to work effectively, each of the elements has to work together. In the NHS these elements are often 'owned' by

Table 23.1 Staffing variations in 'stroke units'

Staff group	Min. per bed	Max. per bed	Variation
Nurses	0.80	1.92	190%
Occupational therapists	0.03	0.13	433%
Physiotherapists	0.07	0.26	371%
Speech and language therapists	0.02	0.07	350%

different organizations. It was extremely rare to find anyone in the visited districts with a clear responsibility for the 'big picture', i.e. a stroke service view for the whole population. It was also found that there was no simple mechanism of obtaining a primary care view on the nature of the community aspects of a stroke service, other than through secondary care leadership. The net result was that apart from isolated examples from enthusiastic GPs, there were no significant primary care stroke services beyond the individual GP service.

In conclusion, stroke services are developing in most districts in the UK but the developments are not uniform, even within single districts. Secondary care services are much more developed than primary care. The major concern I have is that the services appear to be designed and then the population fitted in (or not). If service quality is to progress there is a need to design services on a population, not an organizational, basis. Furthermore, services will need to be more explicit on the dis-benefits of interventions if patients are to be advised appropriately. Finally, the major challenge for the future is to devise ways of assessing systems of care as well as single interventions within single organizations.

References

1. (1990). *The Concise Oxford Dictionary* (8th edn). Oxford University Press, Oxford.
2. Lohr, K. (ed.) (1990). *Medicare: A Strategy for Quality Assurance, Vol. 1.* National Academy Press, Washington, DC.
3. Clinical Standards Advisory Group (1998). *Report on clinical effectiveness using stroke care as an example.* The Stationery Office, London.
4. Checkland, P. B. (1971). A systems map of the universe. *J. Syst. Eng.,* **2,** 2.
5. Checkland, P. (1993). *Systems thinking, systems practice.* John Wiley, Chichester.
6. Wilson, B. (1990). Systems, concepts, methodologies, and applications. John Wiley, Chichester.
7. Stroke Unit Trialists' Collaboration (1997). Collaborative systematic review of the randomised trials of organised in-patient (stroke unit) care after stroke. *Br. Med. J.,* **314,** 1151–9.
8. NHS Executive (1998). *The new NHS, modern and dependable: A national framework for assessing performance* [consultation document]. NHSE, Leeds.
9. Davenport, R. J., Dennis, M. S., Warlow, C. P. (1996). Effect of correcting outcome data for case-mix: An example from stroke medicine. *Br. Med. J.,* **312,** 1503–5.
10. Atrial Fibrillation Investigators (1994). Risk factors for stroke and efficacy of antithrombotic therapy in atrial fibrillation. *Arch. Intern. Med.,* **154,** 1449–55.

11. European Atrial Fibrillation Trial (EAFT) Study Group (1993). Secondary prevention in non-rheumatic atrial fibrillation after transient ischaemic attack or minor stroke. *Lancet*, **342**, 1255–62.
12. Wickramsinge, L. S. P., Basu, S. K., Bansal, S. K. (1988). Long-term oral anticoagulant therapy in elderly patients. *Age Ageing*, **17**, 388–96.
13. Landefield, C. S., Beyth, R. J. (1993). Risk for anticoagulant-related bleeding: A meta-analysis. *Am. J. Med.*, **95**, 315–28.
14. Lundstrom, T., Ryde'n, L. (1989). Haemorrhagic and thrombotic complications in patients with atrial fibrillation on anticoagulation prophylaxis. *J. Int. Med.*, **225**, 137–42.
15. Gustafsson, C., Asplund, K., Britton, M., Norrving, B., Olsson, B., Marke, L. A. (1992). Cost-effectiveness of primary stroke prevention in atrial fibrillation. Swedish national perspective. *Br. Med. J.*, **305**, 1457–60.

24 Comparing outcomes of stroke services in Europe

DR CHARLES WOLFE*

*Reader in Public Health Medicine, Guy's, King's, and
St Thomas' Hospitals School of Medicine, London*

Background

Over 400 000 people die as a result of stroke each year in Western Europe. There are significant variations in mortality from stroke in Europe.[1] The MONICA (Monitoring Cardiovascular Diseases) study of stroke incidence demonstrated large differences in stroke incidence and case fatality around Europe. A survey of consultant opinion in the UK demonstrated that well organized stroke services are patchy and haphazard, and audits of stroke care in the United Kingdom have identified poor adherence to stroke guidelines. These types of variation in incidence, management, and survival have to be borne in mind when considering the guidelines the European Stroke Council has set for stroke services in the millennium and how they can be achieved in such diverse settings.[2]

Methods

Study centres

A European Union BIOMED Concerted Action was initiated to establish the relationships between resource use, costs, and outcome of different packages of care for stroke.[3] The project has involved 12 centres (22 hospitals) in seven European countries, namely England, France, Germany, Hungary, Italy, Portugal, and Spain. The hospitals are not necessarily typical of care in their country, but they provide general acute care and some are also teaching hospitals.

*On behalf of the European Union BIOMED Study of Stroke Care Group.

Data collection

Hospital-based registers were established in September 1993 for one calendar year to collect patient-based data prospectively. Data collection related to first-ever stroke admissions using the World Health Organization definition and well-validated case-mix variables were collected by dedicated data collectors in each centre.[4]

Baseline information used for these analyses included demographic factors (i.e. age, sex, pre-stroke-modified Rankin score, living conditions prior to stroke); clinical state, including risk factors, at the time of maximum impairment (level of consciousness, site of paralysis/weakness, speech or swallowing problems as a result of stroke, incontinence); type of stroke (cerebral infarction or haemorrhage, subarachnoid haemorrhage); use of hospital resources (type of bed, e.g. medical, neurological, intensive care, surgery, rehabilitation, private, other; length of stay in hospital); use of major diagnostic tests (brain imaging, angiography, carotid Doppler); and major therapeutic interventions (neurosurgery).

Three-month data

The living conditions at three months were noted (alone, with companion, institutionalized). The clinical state was reassessed in an identical manner to the initial assessment. The use of further major diagnostic tests (brain imaging, angiography, carotid Doppler, echocardiogram), rehabilitation, and visits to the physician/family doctor were documented. Outcome was assessed in terms of survival to three months (including whether stroke was the cause of death) and disability (Barthel and modified Rankin scales).

Results

A total of 4537 first-ever strokes were registered in the 12 centres. The loss to follow-up rates varied from 0–35%, with six centres having loss to follow-up rates of less than 10%. The mean age of the entire cohort was 72 years (SD 12.05), with a minimum of 14 and maximum of 94, and with significant variation between centres ($p < 0.001$). A total of 2275 (50.14%) were female, with significant differences in the proportion of each sex between centres ($p = 0.014$).

There were significant differences between centres for all case-mix variables ($p < 0.001$ in all cases) which probably reflected different admission policies in the various types of units. There were also obvious differences between centres in the use of medical and neurological beds. The length of stay in the acute hospital setting ranged from 11 days in Portugal to 37 days in inner London. The use of brain imaging also varied significantly, ranging from 30% in a UK centre to 97% in France.

At three months the proportion of patients living at home alone ranged from 7% in Hungary to 57% in Spain. The crude comparisons of outcome varied significantly between centres and hence adjustment for case-mix was undertaken using multinomial logistic regression modelling techniques. The results of these analyses showed that the predicted death rate for the initial 4537 patients would range from 19% if they were all treated in the French centres to 42% if they were treated in one of the English centres.

Discussion

This large European study has described significant differences in three-month outcome in terms of death or dependency for stroke which are unexplained by conventional case-mix variable adjustment. The UK centres also appear to have consistently worse outcomes than the rest of Europe.

There were significant differences in initial stroke severity between units, indicating either different hospital admission policies with some centres catering for more severe strokes or differences in the subtypes of stroke in each area. These variations in case-mix make adjustment essential when comparing outcomes. There are significant differences in the length of stay, type of bed used, and use of brain imaging.

For the majority of patients who did not lose consciousness the study shows significant differences in death and dependency unexplained by case-mix in these 12 centres, and the size of the difference is unlikely to be explained by chance, bias, and confounding. This is a real effect but perhaps not all possible confounding variables have been controlled for.

Variations in mortality and morbidity rates for certain conditions between centres and countries are well documented and used by health care planners and politicians either to set targets for their reduction or to conduct a confidential enquiry to explore the reasons for high rates and consequently improve health care delivery. The *Health of the Nation* White Paper in England set a target for a 40% reduction in mortality rates from stroke by the year 2000, but with very little evidence that the health interventions for people once they had suffered a stroke could alter case fatality. Similarly, the World Health Organization has set targets for the reduction of case fatality for stroke by the year 2005 without indicating what interventions will effectively enable countries and hospitals to achieve these targets.[3]

In conclusion, this study has compiled detailed data on first-ever strokes in 12 centres in Europe and shown, after adjustment for case-mix, significant differences in outcome in patients initially conscious after their stroke. Blackspots within Europe have been identified, but what should be done to improve outcome in these centres remains in doubt. There appears to be room for considerable health gain in certain centres, particularly in the UK. The study cautions against comparisons of this nature which, although leading to further understanding of the relationship between case-mix, resources, and outcome, do not allow rational policy decisions to be made.

References

1. Holland, W. W. (Project director.) (1991). *European Community atlas of avoidable death*. Oxford University Press, Oxford.
2. World Health Organization (1995). *Pan European Consensus Meeting on Stroke Management*. Helsingborg. Sweden, November 1995.
3. Beech, R., Ratcliffe, M., Tilling, K., Wolfe, C. (1996). Hospital services for stroke care: A European perspective. *Stroke*, 27, 1958–64.
4. Wolfe, C. D. A., Tilling, K., Beech, R., Rudd, A. G. (1999). Variations in case fatality and dependency from stroke in Western and Central Europe. *Stroke*, 30, 350–6.

25   Trends in stroke and its management in Japan

Secretary General of the Japan Stroke Association
Department of Internal Medicine, Osaka National Hospital

Trends

Stroke was the leading cause of death in Japan between 1951 and 1980, but has since dropped to second and now third place. This is largely attributable to the decrease of death due to cerebral haemorrhage. In 1997, approximately 139 000 people died of stroke, representing 15.2% of total deaths. The mortality rates due to infarction, intracerebral haemorrhage (ICH), and subarachnoid haemorrhage (SAH) were 69.2, 26.2, and 11.7 per 100 000 respectively.

A Japanese collaborative study of stroke incidence,[1] conducted from 1975 to 1979 and which covered 20 regional and occupational populations, reported the annual incidence of stroke to be 3.94 for men and 2.52 for women (per 1000 population, aged 40–69). The incidence rates for infarction in men and women were 1.87 and 1.10, respectively. Incidence rates for ICH were 1.26 and 0.59. Regarding the subtype of stroke, lacunar infarction and ICH were more frequently found than in the US, which corresponds to between one-third to one-half and one-fifth of stroke, respectively.[2] The incidence rates of both infarction and ICH have decreased since the 1960s. A community study in Hisayama[3] showed that annual incidence rates for infarction decreased, falling from 8.7 (men) and 6.0 (women) per 1000 people in 1961–66 to 7.0 and 3.1 in 1972–76. Those for ICH decreased from 3.1 (men) and 0.7 (women) to 2.0 and 0.6, respectively.

Despite declining incidence rates of infarction and ICH, the number of stroke patients in Japan has increased, reaching 1.7 million in 1996. One-year survival was reported to be approximately 70%.[4] Among survivors, about half are independent in activities of daily living one year after stroke. Socially, 40% of the bedridden elderly and home-nurse clients are stroke survivors. In 1996, 8.1% of medical expenditures were used for stroke.

Recently, the effectiveness of a community-based hypertension control programme for decreasing stroke incidence, especially in men, was shown in a study in north-eastern Japan.[5] Stroke incidence declined more in the full-intervention community than in the minimal-intervention community. This study suggests the importance of public campaigns for the prevention of stroke.

Management

At present, no precise data on stroke management are available in Japan. In 1998, a retrospective survey by postal inquiry was begun by Yamaguchi, *et al.*, and a prospective survey was scheduled to begin in 1999. A preliminary report from the retrospective survey of 4948 major medical facilities gives a snapshot of current conditions – out of 4948 facilities, 2034 departments in 1777 facilities responded. Of the respondents, 49% treated more than 50 stroke patients per year, 36% treated more than 50 infarction patients, 10% treated 50+ ICH patients, and 3% treated 50+ SAH patients annually. Stroke patients were treated by neurosurgeons, internists, neurologists, cardiologists, etc. The average number of beds for stroke was 23. Three per cent used stroke units, 24% used intensive care units, and 73% used neither. In 6% of the hospitals that responded, more than 75% of infarction patients were treated within six hours after onset. As an acute therapy for ischaemic stroke, sodium ozagrel, a TXA_2 synthetase inhibitor, was used in 87% and argatroban, a selective antithrombotic drug, was used in 52% of the responding facilities. Surgical treatments, mainly decompression, were used for acute infarction in 14% of the facilities. In 78% of the hospitals, the mean length of hospital stay was more than four weeks.

The Japan Stroke Association

Inaugurated in 1997, the Japan Stroke Association (JSA) aims at prevention of stroke and support for stroke survivors and their families. The main activities are publication of newsletters and leaflets, providing monthly telephone counselling, organizing stroke symposia for citizens, and conducting surveys.

Three survey projects were started in 1998: (a) an analysis of enquiries made to the telephone consultation service of JSA, (b) a survey concerning people's awareness of stroke, and (c) a survey of how stroke patients seek medical treatment and how they are treated.

The telephone consultation project ran for nine months from January 1998, during which 240 people made 276 enquiries to the Association. Half of the enquirers were persons who were concerned, mainly aged between 55–74. Eighty per cent of the questions involved medical information, especially on the sequelae (35.9%) and prevention (15.9%) of stroke. These figures suggest a significant need for medical information among stroke survivors, their families, and the general public.

The survey concerning stroke awareness questioned people about symptoms, risk factors, what to do at the onset of symptoms, and their image of stroke as an illness. The subjects were from the general public, including high-school and university students, workers, the elderly, and people concerned with medical/welfare services, including home helpers, nurses, and medical doctors. Preliminary results from the 154 high-school students, 69 university (non-medical) students, and 125 elderly showed that only 30% could name at least one stroke symptom, and only 43% could name at least one risk factor correctly. Ninety-seven per cent understood that stroke needs rapid response. Only 4% named stroke as the most important disease in Japan, while cancer and AIDS were named by 75% and 9%, respectively.

Conclusion

Considering the significant impact of stroke on Japanese society and individuals, further prevention should be achieved using community intervention. As to its management in Japan, efforts to monitor the present situation have just been initiated.

References

1. Komachi, Y., Tanaka, H., Shimamoto, T., *et al*. (1984). A collaborative study of stroke incidence in Japan. *Stroke*, **15**, 28–36.
2. Fujishima, M. (1996). Cerebrovascular disorders among the Japanese. *J. Jpn. Soc. Intern. Med.*, **85**(9), 1407–18.
3. Ueda, K., Omae, T., Hirota, Y., *et al*. (1981). Decreasing trend in incidence and mortality from stroke in Hisayama residents, Japan. *Stroke*, **12**, 154–60.
4. Kojima, S., Omura, T., Wakamatsu, W., *et al*. (1990). Prognosis and disability of stroke patients after 5 years in Akita, Japan. *Stroke*, **21**, 72–7.
5. Iso, H., Shimamoto, T., Naito, Y., *et. al*. (1998). Effects of a long-term hypertension control programme on stroke incidence and prevalence in a rural community in north-eastern Japan. *Stroke*, **29**, 1510–18.

26 The role of The Stroke Association in research and development

PROFESSOR W. W. HOLLAND

Emeritus Professor of Public Health Medicine, University of London
Chairman of Research and Development Committee, The Stroke Association

The papers that have been presented to The Stroke Association's Centenary International Scientific Conference demonstrate both the breadth and quality of research on stroke. Obviously not all the research described has been supported by the Association, but much of it has.

It is gratifying that the field has expanded so greatly, and that it has attracted so many high-quality researchers. As the introductory lectures by Professors Marshall and Brocklehurst have shown, the interest in stroke is relatively recent and is associated with the development of effective forms of prevention and treatment which have influenced the outcome.

The Association has always supported research in the field, and we are proud of our ability to expand our research support. Several of the major studies which have led to an improvement in stroke prevention, care, and treatment have either been supported initially, in part, or wholly by the Association.

One of our aims has always been to support and fund research by all the disciplines involved in stroke care. We have thus been able to reinforce the essential emphasis that stroke care involves a variety of different disciplines, and that research improves the performance of professionals. As part of our programme we have, for some years, supported training fellowships. These have not been restricted just to medically qualified personnel, but we have supported physiotherapists, occupational therapists, and speech therapists to obtain the necessary formal academic training (MScs and PhDs) so that they can participate in research on an equal footing to medical practitioners. Several of the speakers and participants at this meeting have benefited from this programme.

As a result of the growth and quality of researchers in stroke, the Association funds a Chair in Stroke Medicine at Nottingham

University, a stroke therapy research unit at Manchester, and a lecturer in stroke medicine in relation to Afro-Caribbeans at King's College, London.

We now usually receive about 100 applications for research grants each year. The quality of these applications has improved considerably in the past five or so years but unfortunately we are only able to fund about 10% of those who apply. In addition, the Association has reviewed the current research findings and identified the areas of greatest need.[1] This has been widely circulated and, as a result, we have embarked on funding two programme grants each year. The area identified as being of highest priority was the prevention of stroke; two programme grants were awarded for this last year. This year we will be funding two programmes for studies on stroke amongst Afro-Caribbeans and other ethnic minority groups who have a particularly high incidence and poor outcome. Next year we will fund two studies on the psychological consequences (and treatment) of stroke.

In addition to funding original research we also support, and evaluate, service developments shown to be necessary from research findings. Thus we have helped to fund the appointment of stroke physicians responsible for the coordination of stroke services in eight districts to serve as models of what can and should be done. We have also supported six groups, in different parts of the UK, to develop community rehabilitation services. These are being formally evaluated by a unit in Leeds in order that we can learn how best to deliver such services.

Although we are very satisfied by the work of those we support, we cannot rest on our laurels. One of our tasks is to stimulate and support work amongst groups involved in stroke. It is disappointing that both the quantity and quality of research proposals from nursing and primary care (general practitioners) has not been as great as that of other professional groups.

The lack of good research proposals or interest by general practitioners in introducing innovative schemes of community care for stroke is particularly worrying in view of their vital role in caring for this group. Although we are trying to rectify this deficit, we cannot act alone – I hope that the Royal College of General Practitioners will become involved and stimulate the field to promote worthwhile research.

There have recently been three major reviews of the services provided for stroke: the Clinical Standards Advisory Group investigation described by Professor Martin Severs, the study by Professor Shah

Ebrahim which was a repeat of one done four years ago, and the Royal College of Physicians' multidisciplinary audit of stroke, the complete results of which have not yet been published.

In 1983, a group of us first published a geographical analysis of standardized mortality ratios for the years 1974–79 of what we termed 'avoidable deaths'.[2] Stroke and hypertension mortality in those aged less than 65 years was one of the 12 categories we included. We demonstrated a greater than threefold variation in mortality between the best and the worst area. Subsequently this analysis was repeated for two further quinquennia, i.e. 1980–84 and 1985–89, and included in the European Community Atlas of Avoidable Death.[3] There has been a fall in mortality from stroke in all areas, but the variation between areas persists. The studies of Wolfe and his colleagues have shown that we are not as good in the care of patients with stroke as some of our European colleagues. The findings of Severs, Ebrahim, and the Royal College audit show that there are major variations in the organization and processes of stroke care in England. This has been known for more than two years to have a major impact in reducing mortality and residual disability.

These findings link research to practice. Research has led the way in exploring better ways to prevent and treat stroke. It is encouraging that this has been applied in some places but it is disappointing that at least half of the population of England still does not receive better organized care, which costs no more and may even cost less than the haphazard care practised for so long. It is, however, encouraging that some of the areas we identified as having very high mortality rates 10–20 years ago now appear to be providing good hospital care, as shown by the Royal College of Physicians' audit study.

These findings also pose major research challenges. How can we improve preventive services in the community and apply the known, effective measures more widely; what components of stroke care actually make a difference in mortality and disability; and how can we improve both treatment and rehabilitation?

The Association spends about £2.5 million per annum on research and development, more than half its income from donations. We are not the only group to support research, but are probably the major single source. From the applications we receive and from the priorities we have identified, we could probably easily spend twice as much. Due to changes in government, university, and Medical Research Council policies for the funding and accountability of research and health services, the increase in research applications has been accompanied by a rise in the costs of research. This is partly due to the precise attribution of the costs of research so that expenditures have to be clearly identified as research costs and not included in general NHS, university, etc. expenditures, and partly by the rising costs of staff, equipment, and materials.

The current preoccupation with 'evidence-based medicine' has also meant that the gold standard of the randomized controlled trial is considered essential before changes in treatment or health policy are introduced. Unfortunately these trials usually need to be of very large size in order to show the effects that are likely to occur in the treatment of stroke. Thus they are very expensive and it is difficult to provide support from the limited resources we have available. For the future it is crucial to consider alternative ways of answering the real questions of the effectiveness of changes in treatment without the disadvantages of expensive controlled trials able to answer only limited questions in an experimental mode, without necessarily being applicable to the clinical situation. This is a major challenge for the research community and one that would have been relished by my teacher, Austin Bradford Hill, who was responsible for the introduction of randomized controlled trails to clinical medicine in the UK.

I hope that The Stroke Association's Centenary International Scientific Conference, and the celebrations of its centenary, will influence those responsible for the delivery of services to rectify the unacceptable variations in the provision of effective services, and will also lead to an increase in funds for stroke services and research and thus to a better outcome for people affected by stroke.

References

1. Wolf, C., Rudd, A., Beech, R. (ed.) (1996). *Stroke services and research: An overview, with recommendations for future research.* The Stroke Association, London.
2. Charlton, J. R. H., Hartley, R. M., Silver, R., Holland, W. W. (1983). Geographical variation in mortality from conditions amenable to medical intervention in England and Wales. *Lancet*, 1, 691.
3. Holland, W. W. *European Community atlas of avoidable death.* CEC Health Services Research Series No. 3 and ibid. (1991) Series No. 6 (2nd edn) and ibid. (1997) Series No. 9. Oxford University Press, Oxford.
4. Stroke Unit Trialists' Collaboration (1997). Collaborative systematic review of the randomised trails of organised in-patient (stroke unit) care after stroke. *Br. Med. J.*, 914, 1151–9.

27   A hundred years of stroke research

PROFESSOR J. VAN GIJN

*Professor of Neurology University
Department of Neurology, Utrecht, The Netherlands*

Stroke is not a single condition. Inevitably more and more subdivisions are recognized as time goes on. I shall limit my historical overview to the three main categories of stroke:

(a) occlusion of a blood vessel in the brain (cerebral infarction or ischaemic stroke, 80%);
(b) rupture of a blood vessel within the brain tissue (intracerebral haemorrhage, 15%);
(c) rupture of a bulge (aneurysm in a blood vessel at the undersurface of the brain, in the fluid-filled space between the brain membranes – subarachnoid haemorrhage, 5%).

The term 'apoplexy' was first used by the ancient Greek physician, Hippocrates, and encompassed all forms of stroke. In the second half of this century it became synonymous with 'intracerebral haemorrhage', and now it has fallen into disuse. An equally antiquated term is 'cerebrovascular accident', which actually means nothing more than 'stroke'. It was once favoured by physicians too shy to try and make further distinctions, or too lofty to share words with the laity.

At the beginning of the 20th century some important steps towards the understanding of stroke had already been made. Cerebral infarction ('softening' of the brain), more difficult to recognize than intracerebral bleeding, had been identified as a separate kind of stroke in 1823 (by Léon Rostan, in Paris). In Berlin, Rudolf Virchow (1821–1902), pathologist and also social reformer, found that occlusion of arteries was mostly caused by abnormalities of the vessel wall – and not of the blood, as had been previously supposed. In addition, he found that a blood clot formed on the damaged wall of an artery, or on a damaged heart valve, could be dislodged and carried away until it occluded a smaller artery downstream ('embolism'). Subarachnoid haemorrhage had been first described in the UK, in

1812, by Cheyne ('meningeal apoplexy'), and one year later Blackall pointed out the ruptured aneurysm; yet all such observations had only been made after death.

In the course of the 20th century our understanding of the different types of stroke has grown further, and – more important – in the second half of that period methods of treatments evolved from which patients really stood to gain.

Cerebral infarction

As early as 1905 Chiari drew attention to the frequency of atherosclerotic lesions of the carotid artery in the neck, at the site where it bifurcates into the internal carotid artery (to the brain) and the external carotid artery (to the face). Yet it took several more decades for the ingrained notion of 'brain thrombosis' to be driven from the average physician's mind. In fact, atherosclerosis of the large vessels within the brain is very rare, at least in the Western world.

Two main factors were important in changing the medical mindset from 'thrombosis' to 'embolism' – not only from the heart, but also from arteries upstream. The first was the advent of cerebral angiography by the Portuguese neurosurgeon, Egas Moniz, in 1927. This method made it possible to visualize the arteries in the neck – and their abnormalities – by the injection of an iodinated contrast substance into the arteries (iodine has high absorption values for X-rays, which had been discovered in 1895 by Roentgen). This made it possible to identify narrowing or occlusion of the carotid artery. Yet direct puncture of the artery in the neck had its complications, and angiography became common only after 1953 when Seldinger (in Sweden) described a method to introduce a long catheter via an artery in the groin. The method is now being replaced by less invasive or even non-invasive methods (spiral CT scanning, magnetic resonance angiography).

The second factor, almost coinciding with the advent of modern angiography, was formed by some of the work of the neurologist, C. Miller Fisher, a born Canadian, in Boston in the 1950s. To begin with, he again drew attention to lesions at the carotid bifurcation in autopsy studies. Moreover, he correlated these lesions with clinical features – not only with paralysis of the face, arm, and leg on the other side of the body (corresponding with the same side of the brain), but also with fleeting attacks of blindness in the eye on the same side. Together with increased recognition of fleeting attacks in which there was dysfunction not of the eye but of certain parts of the brain (e.g. paralysis of limbs, or loss of language abilities), this led to the notion of stroke warnings ('transient ischaemic attacks' or TIAs). In the past such attacks had been attributed to sudden narrowing ('spasm') of a blood vessel, or to low blood pressure, but now they came to be regarded as often being caused by small blood clots that had broken off from an atherosclerotic patch (plaque) in the internal carotid artery. If the clot was small, or if it easily broke up in small fragments, the result was a TIA. If not, the result was a stroke – always incapacitating, often devastating.

These insights at last led to treatments that were effective; that is, to some extent. The example of the first recorded carotid endarterectomy, by Eastcott and others in 1954, was being followed by a rapidly increasing number of vascular surgeons, for a variety of indications, until counter-reactions emphasized the dangers of the operation. Charles Warlow (UK) and later Henry Barnett (Canada) were instrumental in solving this problem, in the 1980s, through the methods of the controlled clinical trial (first devised in 1948 by Austin Bradford Hill for the MRC streptomycin trial of pulmonary tuberculosis). These two trials made clear that some patients benefit from the operation (especially that the degree of narrowing matters), whereas others do not.

Medical treatment should start with primary prevention, by modification of risk factors such as blood pressure and smoking. More specific, of course, is secondary prevention after a patient has had a stroke or a stroke warning. A necessary step was the advent of CT scanning, in the 1970s, which made it possible to distinguish with certainty between haemorrhage and infarction. The era of antiplatelet agents was heralded by the Canadian aspirin trial in 1978 (Henry Barnett). For patients in atrial fibrillation (a common disorder of heart rhythm), another European trial has taught us that anticoagulants are beneficial. Finally, the mid-1990s saw the advent of thrombolysis for acute stroke in the wake of similar treatments for myocardial infarction. The gain is still modest, and we are not yet quite sure for whom, but at least we have a foot in the door.

Intracerebral haemorrhage

This story has a much less optimistic note. Most improvements in outcome result from better general medical care, such as the prevention of bedsores and infection. Surgical treatment is regularly

128   *Stroke: past, present, and future*

performed in many centres, but no evidence exists from clinical trials that evacuation of a large clot in the brain is beneficial in terms of quality-adjusted life years.

Subarachnoid haemorrhage

If patients survive the initial episode they are threatened by several secondary complications, of which rebleeding is the most feared. In population-based studies the case fatality rate is still around 50%, with a small but definite improvement over time. It was not until the 1920s that the diagnosis was made during life (Charles Symonds, 1923). Again, catheter angiography (after 1953) made it possible to identify the aneurysm. Diagnosis has been facilitated even more by CT scanning, which points at the origin of the haemorrhage.

The Edinburgh neurosurgeon, Norman Dott, performed the first operation on a patient with a ruptured aneurysm in 1931. Of course he did not know beforehand where it exactly was; after he had found it he wound pieces of muscle around it. Improved diagnosis paved the way for surgical intervention on a wider scale. The operation now most often consists of putting a metal clip on the weak bulge in the artery. The latest development, which might well replace most operations, is endovascular occlusion, a method in which the radiologist uses a catheter technique to put small metal coils in the aneurysm until it is occluded.

This is where we were in 1999. Stroke is no longer the Cinderella of medicine. Where some treatments have proved to work, others are bound to arrive. Many young and gifted physicians dedicate their research efforts to stroke. Rehabilitation after stroke, still in its infancy, may hold unsuspected promise. But all these professionals cannot succeed without the help of society in general, and of volunteers in particular.

Further reading

Hachinski, V. M. (1982). Transient cerebral ischemia: a historical sketch. In: *Historical aspects of the neurosciences (Festschrift for M. Critchley)* (ed. F. Clifford Rose, W. F. Bynum), pp. 185–93. Raven Press, New York.
Ljunggren, B., Sharma, S., Buchfelder, M. (1993). Intracranial aneurysms. *Neurosurg. Quart.*, 3, 120–52.
McHenry, L. C. (1981). A history of stroke. *Int. J. Neurol.*, 15, 314–26.

Schiller, F. (1970). Concepts of stroke before and after Virchow. *Med. Hist.*, **14**, 115–31.

Warlow, C. P., Dennis, M. S., van Gijn, J., Hankey, G. J., Sandercock, P. A. G., Bamford, J. M., *et al.* (1996). *Stroke: A practical guide to management.* Blackwell Science, Oxford.

Index